DO IT TODAY

More from Darius Foroux

Win Your Inner Battles (2016)

How To Go From Procrastinate Hero to Procrastinate Zero (2016)

THINK STRAIGHT (2017)

What It Takes To Be Free (2019)

Highly Productive Remote Work (2020)

The Road to Better Habits, Updated and Expanded (2021)

Find them all at **dariusforoux.com/books**

Do It Today

Overcome Procrastination, Improve
Productivity, and Achieve More
Meaningful Things

Written by

DARIUS FOROUX

ISBN: 9781983184529

About The Author

Darius Foroux (pronounced as Da-reeus Fo-roo) is the author of 7 books, and the creator of 6 online courses. He writes about productivity, business, and wealth building. His ideas and work have been featured in TIME, NBC, Fast Company, Inc., Observer, and many more publications. Until now, more than 30 million people have read his articles.

Thank You: A Gift

Thank you for purchasing this book. I really appreciate that you picked this book out of the millions of options you have. Deciding to read one book over the other might seem small to a reader with so many options, but to me, the author, it means everything.

To show you my gratitude, I want to offer you something in return. I've put together a bundle of 6 resources with proven tips for optimizing your life and work.

It's called The Growth Kit and it includes 4 short eBooks, a checklist, and an infographic.

Go to dariusforoux.com/growth-kit to grab your free kit.

Enjoy!

-Darius

Table Of Contents

Preface

Thanks for taking the time to read this book. You could've done a million other things with your time, yet you decided to pick up this book about improving your productivity. When I published the first edition of this book in 2018, the economy was doing well, and more people were excited about online opportunities than ever. As I'm writing this new preface, it's four years later, and we're living in a totally different world.

The 2020s decade started with a pandemic, then we got extraordinary inflation, a war in Europe, and conflicts between the two super-powers of the world, and it seems like there is no end to these global challenges. All of these things impact our lives. But there's another, bigger, challenge we're going through in our modern lives. We're getting more passive. So many of us live on auto-pilot. The pressure of daily life is so high that we're only doing the bare minimum just to survive.

But what happened to "thriving" in the world? What happened to getting the most out of yourself? In our strange world, which is both complex and also filled with many temptations, it's easy to forget yourself. But we can't allow that to happen. We must take control of our time, actions, and attention. Only then can we truly thrive.

That's what Do It Today is all about. This book gives you the tools to adapt and thrive in today's fast-paced world. And the best thing? You can improve your productivity, boost focus, and overcome procrastination without sacrificing your mental health. Yes, that's possible. You CAN be a person who gets a lot done and you can be happy at the same time. It's a myth that you need to be a miserable workaholic to achieve results in your life. Based on the feedback I've received from readers of Do It Today over the past several years, I can confidently say that this book will help you. This book's print and digital editions have sold over 60,000 copies worldwide. And I've received more than a thousand emails from readers who said this book changed their life. Isn't that weird?

Something so simple as a book has the ability to change everything. I can relate to that 100%. In fact, that's why I started writing. For years, I tried to find a breakthrough and change my life. I wanted what so many of us are after: A good life, a career I enjoy, doing fun things, earning good money, and spending time with great people. I just didn't know how to make that happen until I discovered personal development books.

Do It Today is a movement. A philosophy. A way of life.

The title didn't have a profound meaning when I first wrote this book. I had written an article called Do It Today, which I thought captured my philosophy for life nicely. But I didn't give the title much thought. Lately, I've been repeating the phrase Do It Today to myself while doing hard work. Today I went on an intense ride on my road bike, and towards the end of the one-hour workout, I repeated the phrase to myself.

Do It Today, as in, get the most out of your workout right

now. Leave it all on the table. Don't think, "I have to work tomorrow," or anything else that you might use as an excuse not to push yourself. My mind tries to do that all the time.

Take writing this new preface. I've been thinking about writing this all week. Sometimes we need to repeat the phrase Do It Today multiple times before we actually do it that day. But that's good. At least this is a motto that helps you to do meaningful work.

Do It Today is a lifestyle. I've been living this lifestyle for many years, but I finally have a name for it. If you don't have a motto for life, I invite you to adopt this one. Say it to yourself when you're getting ready for work. Say it when you want to work out but don't feel like leaving the house. Share it with your partner when hanging out at home for too long. Talk about it with your co-workers and inspire each other to get more done in less time.

Use the hashtag #DoItToday on social media when you post about the things you're doing in life. Whatever helps you to embody the philosophy of this book. It's truly a lifestyle, and one that's not only rewarding but also good for your health, career, and relationships. Everybody likes someone who does what they say!

I can honestly go on about the benefits of books forever. But let's get down to the actual book. For the past few days, I spent several hours to re-read the book after all this time to see whether it needed updating. But honestly, the content is more relevant today than in 2018. In fact, improving your productivity and overcoming procrastination will be one of the most important things of the 2020s decade. The opportunities are endless if we can improve our output and stay sane. I hope everything inside this book will change your life just like mine. Enjoy!

-Darius

About This Book

As I'm writing this, I'm blocked from accessing my email provider that I use to send out my weekly newsletter. This email provider is the most important service I use to run my blog. It's equally important as my blog itself.

The reason I can't access my email provider and send emails to my subscribers (even new subscribers who join my newsletter are not receiving my welcome email) is that I'm being "list-bombed." It happens when spammers bomb your email list signups with emails from people who didn't want to sign up for your list. And now, I'm known as a spammer because I send emails to people who didn't sign up for them. At least, this is what a website that lists spammers says.

In their eyes, I'm a spammer. Am I one? Of course not. I have a life. However, publishing weekly articles and staying in touch with my readers is also a part of my life. And that's been taken away from me now. The irony is that I migrated to this provider ten days ago. I've spent dozens of hours on that process.

Normally, I would get pissed off about this situation and start blaming someone. After all, I invested a lot of time in building a large email list. And for a moment, I did get upset about being blocked from it. But you know what I did next? I started doing something else that's important. I started this book.

Just like that. I moved on to the next thing. Life doesn't stop. And every single second, we're getting closer to death. I must say, three years ago, I was far away from the person that I am today. I would complain, feel sorry for myself, blame others, and I would never have acted on anything meaningful. But through reading, journaling, and blogging every week, I have transformed my life.

Like a sculptor, I shaped my philosophy for life during that period. My philosophy can be summarized in three words, and it's the title of this book: *Do it today.* Look, I don't have to tell you that life is finite, and that time is not replenishable.

Every second we invest in something is time that we can never get back. But I want to challenge you to look at the bigger picture.

What you do today determines where you will be in a year, two years, and even ten years from now. Every single day, we keep on doing things that we don't desire. I'm not talking about paying the bills or cleaning your toilet. I'm talking about how you invest the majority of your time. The time that sums up your *life*.

When I was 13 or 14 years old, I watched the movie *Fight Club* for the first time together with one of my friends. One line has been engraved on my mind ever since that moment: "You are not your job, you're not how much money you have in the bank."

I'm glad I watched that movie back then. I've watched the movie more than a dozen times, and I've read the book more than once. That single thought inspired me to become independent. I'm not my job. And I'm certainly not my bank account.

But who are we, if we are not those things?

For the past 17 or 18 years, I've been meditating on that question. As of now, I believe that we are our *actions*. And our actions reveal our character. That's who we are.

The funny thing is that we *are* our job. After all, we spend the majority of our time earning a living. We trade time for money. Whether you like it or not, you have to spend a part of your life doing that. Most people end up trading time for money during their entire life. But a few of us spend their time in a way *now*, that they have a better life *tomorrow*.

That's why I always do it today—especially the important things like:

- Reading
- Exercising
- Investing
- Saving
- Spending time with people I love
- Laughing
- Booking a holiday
- Enjoying my life

And yes, even paying the bills. No matter what happens, I do the *important* things today—not tomorrow.

Find Out What's Important To You

This book is not about life hacks, productivity tips, or any other tactics. We all know about those things. Sure, now and then I share tactical advice that I've applied to achieve more in less time. However, this book contains a collection of articles that I handpicked to help you get more clarity in life.

The recipe for a good life is simple: Get clear on what you want and eliminate everything else from your life. The process is simple, yet it took me many years to figure those things out.

And this book is my journey. Sure, you can find the articles in this book on my blog, but they are not presented in the right order. A blog is organic. I write about the challenges that I face. But with a book, I can give you a structured body of work that serves a specific purpose.

Do It Today is my path and blueprint for overcoming the endless procrastination, improving my productivity, and getting more meaningful things done. And it can be yours too.

How This Book Is Constructed

There are three parts to this journey. In Part I, we start with changing the way we look at life. No more procrastination. No more feeling sorry. No more regrets.

You know, my grandmother was ill for the last few years of her life. She went on and on about the things she didn't do in life. Sure, she talked about the good things too. But the regret was more powerful. Research even shows that negative emotions have a bigger impact on our psyche than positive ones.

So, before I show you how to use your time effectively, and get more things done, I want to focus on our mindset. That's what Part I is about: Shifting from a passive state to an active state. By the end of Part I, I hope that you decide to grab life by the head and say, "I'm in charge."

When you're in charge of your life, and therefore your time, it's the perfect moment to get the best bang for your buck. Because that's all that productivity is: An optimum use of time. In Part II, I have collected the articles that show you how to do that. You'll find more than just "do this and you'll boost your productivity" type of ideas. I take a different route to productivity. For example, one of the articles is about reading 100 books in a year. It's not necessarily about productivity, but it does show you how I approach something that's important to me. When you decide you want to do something, you also must have a map that takes you there. In life, we have to make that map. So, when you read the article about reading more books, look at my thinking process. Look at how I go about my challenge. Only then you can apply the strategies to your own life.

Finally, in Part III, I show you how to stay on the path. It's easy to read an article or listen to some advice and apply it for a day. But that's useless. We only make real progress and achieve big things by doing small things every single day. For instance, one of the articles in Part III is about the power of compounding. When you do the little things every day, they add up. And over time, they form big things like a strong body & mind, self-reliance, a large investment portfolio, and so forth. One thing that I've learned about compounding is that you can also compound hurtful things.

When you complain every day, eat junk food, and never

work out, those things add up too. That's how we become miserable. You almost never hear about how one single moment destroyed a person's life. Of course, tragedies happen. But for the majority of us, we simply let life slip away from us. We decide not to do it today. Because "what's the point?" Well, here's the point: Life is good if you know how to live it. The 30 articles that I present in this book, form a system that's unshakeable (I've formatted the articles specially for Kindle, to make them more readable. And I've made several improvements to many articles, based on new lessons I learned and the feedback I've received from readers.)

When you adopt the habits that I write about in this book, you can take on any challenge that life throws at you. You no longer have to wish that life was easier, you're stronger now.

As I write this, the sun is shining, there are no clouds, it's 28 degrees Celsius (82 Fahrenheit), and I'm sitting shirtless behind my desk in my home—listening to the Chilled-Out Electronic playlist on Apple Music. And all I can think is, "life is good."

Let's get started, my friend.

-Darius

June 7, 2018

Leeuwarden, The Netherlands.

How To Read This Book

Before you start, I want to share a few lessons I learned about reading a book—especially a practical one like this.

- There are no rules to reading a book so feel free to read it in any way or order you want.

- Skip the parts that are not relevant to you. No, you don't have to read a book cover to cover.

- Highlight text and take notes to remember more.

- Skimming a book before you read it can be beneficial. I often skim a book, so I can get a better understanding of what I should skip or focus on. Sometimes, I find out that I can't skip anything. Sometimes, I skip half of a book.

- You only need one idea that can change your life. If a book gives you only one good piece of advice, it's already worth your time.

Happy reading.

Part I: Overcoming Procrastination

"You cannot escape the responsibility of tomorrow by evading it today."

- Abraham Lincoln

Do It Today, Not Tomorrow

Every time I put off a decision, hit the snooze button, skipped the gym, or didn't complete my tasks because I didn't feel like it, I always had an explanation for my continual procrastination. I told myself I was tired. Or that it could wait until tomorrow. Who cares if you put off something, right?

Well, you should care.

Because you're the one who's responsible for your life. Too often, we look at productivity tips, apps or tools as the magic answer to our problems. But that also means we allow ourselves to blame external things for our lack of productivity.

- "No, it's not me, it's my old laptop. It sucks, and I can't work this way."
- "The office is too loud."
- "People keep calling and emailing me."
- "I never have time."

Battling procrastination is an inner battle. I have many examples of that in my personal life. In 2013, I felt my career was stuck. Two years before that, I started a company with my dad. But after two years, I became restless because I wanted to do more and learn more.

So I did some freelancing. I built websites, did copywriting, content marketing, and some design work. But it didn't take off. Why? I never did the uncomfortable work. Instead, I found a job to escape those hard tasks.

We all escape at times.

Building a business or career is hard. It requires you to do difficult, tedious, and unsatisfying tasks. If you want more clients or work, no one is going to hand it to you. You have to hustle. Do content marketing, one-on-one sales, network, or whatever method you use to grow your business.

And if you want to climb the corporate ladder, you have to form alliances, be strategic, outperform your targets, and be great at what you do.

That's what you SHOULD do, right? Most of us already know these things. Or, you will find out about it. There's no such thing as a secret to succeeding at work.

However, we prefer to escape work. And that's at the core of procrastination to me.

You know what you have to do, but you don't do it. Instead, you open a news site and start reading useless news items. Or you browse your Instagram feed without liking one picture because you hate your life. Maybe you browse Zara, H&M, Net-A-Porter, Mr. Porter, or whatever online shop you like. That was, and to a degree still is, the story of my life. For example, I'm now working on a new book. I know what it's about and I also have a title. But writing is also very difficult work to me.

So I look for relief. I answer emails, read articles, go for coffee, do some online shopping, and work on recurring tasks to run my business. It's not that I'm disorganized. It's because I'm battling myself. Steven Pressfield calls this inner enemy Resistance in his classic, The War Of Art. And this is what he says about it:

"Resistance is always lying and always full of shit."

Do It Today, Not Tomorrow

I always have to keep reminding myself of that. When you procrastinate, you always want to do it tomorrow. I'm still like that. I think that's hardwired into us. The difference between me now, and three years ago is small but simple: I rely on a system to live a productive, happy, and purposeful life.

Back then I had no idea how to get things done. I always gave up quickly, felt stuck, unhappy, and frustrated. But now, I've found a way to overcome my challenges. Here's how I did it:

- **I exercise my mental toughness every day.** I used to neglect my brain. I was mentally weak, thought too much, and didn't rely on myself. It wasn't because I lacked skills. It was because I didn't trust in my ability to figure things out. So I started reading about Stoicism, Pragmatism and Mindfulness; anything that helps you to control your thoughts and improve your mental toughness. I don't want to be a slave to my thoughts. I want the opposite.

- **I exercise my body every day.** When I don't exercise, I'm restless, lack focus, energy, and confidence. By exercising my brain and body every day, I'm always war-ready. I learned that overcoming procrastination starts before you fight the war. Soldiers don't go to war untrained either, right? Be in great shape, mentally and physically. Always.

- **I have a set of daily habits that help me to be in control of my life.** I journal, read, set daily priorities, and don't consume useless information. I also make sure I interact with my friends and family every day. Human contact is important. This keeps me grounded. I don't have high expectations of life. And I enjoy my days. I never look beyond that.

- **I always have a list of small (but important) tasks that I have to complete.** Let's take my new book for example. I often want to escape difficult things like actually sitting down and writing. So I tell myself today is not a good day. But every time I think that, I open my list of small tasks and work on one of those things TODAY.

- **I study and practice the science of persuasion to get my message across.** My mentor taught me: "You can be the best writer and teacher in the world, but if no one knows about it, you can't make an impact." The science of persuasion helps you to write better pitches, cover letters, website copy, emails, etc.

Of course, it takes time to develop the foundation of this strategy. And there's a lot more to it. But it's not magic. However, it's also not easy to live a productive life. And it's definitely not about technology or hacks. It's about developing a sustainable system to build your life, career, and business on. What's your system for living a productive life?

Whatever it is: Work on it today. Not tomorrow.

What I Do When I Can't Focus

Do you struggle to finish your tasks? Are you always distracted by notifications, gossiping, or anything that's random? In that case, you and I are alike. Because focusing on a single thing is one of the hardest things at work. There's always something that interrupts you, right?

- Another person
- A call
- A meeting
- A false emergency
- Your cat
- A stranger's cat
- News about last night's NBA game

Sure, you can blame those things — but that's weak. You and I both know that those things can't interrupt you without your permission. That means every time you're not focused; you're giving someone or something permission to enter your mind. Scary, isn't it? That's how I look at interruptions. But I have to admit that I can't maintain my focus all the time. Sometimes, I give in. It's not good.

Your life doesn't benefit from gossiping, looking at Instagram 439 times a day, watching 49 YouTube videos, and reading negative news articles.

So, what can you do to improve your focus? Here are 2 things that I always do when I find myself not being able to focus on what matters.

1. Eliminate. Eliminate. Eliminate

Every day, we accumulate stuff. I'm not only talking about the stuff you're buying like clothes, kitchen equipment, house decorations, toys, gadgets, or whatever.

We accumulate ideas. Have you ever thought about that? We're exposed to so many ideas that we adopt some of them, and make them our own. For example, many people have told me to create more YouTube videos. My family, friends, team members, readers, students — everybody has ideas. And they want to help. Likewise, I also share my ideas with others. Ideas about how you can improve your life, career, business, or relationships. We all do it. And there's nothing wrong with that.

It only becomes a problem if you don't filter the input you get from people. So after I heard from people that I should make YouTube videos, I thought to myself "Hey! I should make YouTube videos!" I've been thinking a lot about that for the past six months. And I also invested a lot of time in creating a strategy. "What should my videos be about? Where should I record them? How should I edit them? What music should I use?" I've been working on it a lot. And I recently published a video as well.

The response was positive. There's only one problem: It consumes too much of my time and attention. As a consequence, I can spend less time on writing, podcasting, and creating new courses. And those are exactly the things that I *want* to do. I started a blog for a reason: I love to write, and I'm good at it. Therefore, the work is easier, compared to creating YouTube videos, which I'm not that good at.

Plus, I thoroughly enjoy writing articles, books, and material for my online courses. When the work gets hard, I don't mind. But when I was working on YouTube videos, I got frustrated a lot. And again, my focus and work suffered from it. What did I do when I lacked focus? I asked myself this question:

"What thing(s) should I eliminate to make my life so simple that it's easy to focus?"

In this case, I stopped focusing on YouTube. Elimination is a key strategy that I use for many aspects of my life. We accumulate so much unnecessary baggage throughout the years that we consistently need to eliminate:

- Ideas
- Projects
- Work
- Objects
- And so forth

If you find yourself struggling to focus, try this strategy. Make your life so simple that it's a breeze to live. And let's be honest here. Who wants to live a life that's impossible? Life is already hard enough. Don't make it harder.

2. Think About Past Success

Thinking about past success and happiness stimulates the production of serotonin, a chemical nerve our cells produce.

Serotonin is the key chemical that affects every part of your body. Serotonin plays a huge role in our bodily functions. But it also helps to reduce depression, increase libido, stabilize mood, control sleep, and regulate anxiety. Serotonin also plays a massive role in our general *well-being*. But here's why serotonin matters to your focus. Serotonin also regulates delayed gratification. When your serotonin activity goes down, it can lead to a lack of focus on the long-term. You are less likely to act on your plans.

When you lose focus, there's a big chance that your serotonin activity is low. That's why you are giving into short-term pleasures like going out, drinking, shopping, having sex, watching TV, or anything else that gives you short-term pleasure. To improve your focus, boost your serotonin activity. Research shows that exercise can do that. But something else, that's equally effective, and a lot easier is a simple mind-exercise. All you need to do is remember positive events that happened in the past.

Alex Korb, a neuroscientist at UCLA, and the author of The Upward Spiral, explains why remembering positive events helps you to focus on what matters:

"All you need to do [to increase serotonin levels] is remember positive events that have happened in your life. This simple act increases serotonin production in the anterior cingulate cortex,

which is a region just behind the prefrontal cortex that controls attention."

When serotonin goes up, your focus goes up. Ultimately, that's what you should do. I know that it sounds cheesy, but when something is wrong, you must fix it.

When I can't focus, the first thing I do is to acknowledge that I have a problem that needs a solution. Some people go through life without even acknowledging that they have problems.

- No, it's not normal to check your phone every 2 minutes.
- No, it's not normal to gossip all the time.
- No, it's not normal to be bored.

Focus on your life. Think about what matters to you. Then, do those things and don't get distracted — stay on the path.

Good luck.

How To Beat Procrastination (backed by science)

Procrastination has been around since the start of modern civilization. Historical figures like Herodotus, Leonardo Da Vinci, Pablo Picasso, Benjamin Franklin, Eleanor Roosevelt, and hundreds of others have talked about how procrastination is the enemy of results.

One of my favorite quotes about procrastination is from Abraham Lincoln:

"You cannot escape the responsibility of tomorrow by evading it today."

The funny thing about procrastination is that we all know that it's harmful. Who actually likes to procrastinate? No one enjoys doing that. Me neither. And yet, procrastination was the story of my life. When I was in college, every semester, this would happen:

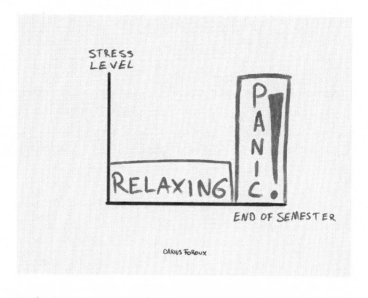

In the beginning of each semester, I was the coolest dude on the planet. Relaxing, going out, enjoying myself. Big time. I experienced no stress whatsoever. However, about a week before my exams, I would freak out.

"Dude, why didn't you begin earlier?" I would tell myself.

And what would follow is an ugly sight of me, with a bunch of Red Bull cans, locked up in my room — freaking out while I was studying. And research shows exactly that: When you procrastinate, you might feel better on the short-term, but you will suffer in the long-term. It doesn't really matter why you procrastinate.

Some love the pressure of deadlines. Some are afraid to fail so they put it off until the very last moment. One thing that all procrastinators have in common is that procrastination has a price.

A highly cited study, published in the American Psychological Society journal, by Dianne Tice and Roy Baumeister discusses the cost of procrastination. It is related to:

- Depression
- Irrational beliefs
- Low self-esteem
- Anxiety
- Stress

Procrastination is not innocent behavior. It's a sign of poor self-regulation. Researchers even compare procrastination to alcohol and drug abuse. It's serious. And I've experienced that for many years.

The years after I got out of college were also a struggle in terms of starting and finishing work. Procrastination is a habit that just sneaks into your system. It's not something you can shake easily. Every time I had a business idea or wanted to start something, it went like this:

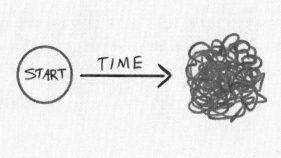

Every time I had an idea or a goal, I would start, but along the way, things would go wrong. I went from start to total chaos. Distractions, other ideas, other opportunities, failure, negative self-talk, etc., would get in the way. And the results are always the same: You never get anything done.

Beating Procrastination

To me, the key finding from the study by Dianne Tice and Roy Baumeister is this:

"The present evidence suggests that procrastinators enjoy themselves rather than working at assigned tasks, until the rising pressure of imminent deadlines forces them to get to work. In this view, procrastination may derive from a lack of self-regulation

and hence a dependency on externally imposed forces to moti-vate work."

Self-regulation, self-control, willpower, are all things that we overestimate. We think: "Yeah sure, I will write a novel in 3 weeks." In our minds, we're all geniuses and mentally strong. But when the work comes, we cop out.

If you're a procrastinator, you can't help but delay work. And that's true for the small and big tasks. Sure, everybody fears to step outside of their comfort zone — that's why we call them comfort zones. It takes courage to make a bold move.

But it sure doesn't take any courage to complete small tasks like paying bills, printing out something for your boss, doing taxes, etc.

The truth is: Procrastination has nothing to do with what you're trying to do — small or big, it can wait until later. It can always wait, right?

For me, completing tasks, went like this:

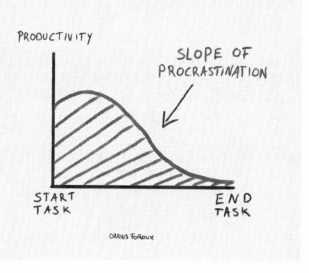

There comes a moment between the start and end of a task—
I call it the slope of procrastination—when you give
into one distraction. And that's exactly the moment you give
up being productive. You start working on a task, you're excited, you're focused, but then, after some time, you think:
Let's read the news for a second.

It always starts with just one thing. Then, you think: I might
as well watch one episode of Game Of Thrones. Then, a
video on YouTube—and then another one. Then, a little bit
of Instagram browsing. And so forth.

It always ends with a bang: **"This is the last time I'm wasting my time!"**

Yeah, right.

Willpower Doesn't Work. Systems Do.

What you really need is a system for doing work. A lot of people shy away from routines, systems and frameworks because they want to have "freedom." I'm sorry to disappoint you: Freedom is your enemy. The fact is that, if you want to get things done, you need rules. What are some things that research proved to be effective?

- Self-imposed deadlines.
- Accountability systems (commitment with friends, or a coach).
- Working/studying in intervals.
- Exercising 30 minutes a day.
- A healthy diet.
- Eliminating distractions.
- **And most importantly: Internal motivation.**

If you combine the right productivity tactics, you have a productivity system. The deadlines create urgency, accountability will create responsibility, working in intervals improves your focus, exercising will give you more energy, so does a healthy diet, and eliminating distractions will take away the temptations.

But there's no system that can help you if you don't have an inner drive. People overcomplicate that concept, but it's simple: Why do you do what you do?

If you don't know. Make something up.

If you know why you're doing something, even the most annoying tasks become bearable. It will become a part of the bigger picture.

So, instead of diving into work, take a step back, think about why you do what you do, and then rely on a system that supports that. Not rocket science. Just science.

How To Stop Wasting Time and Improve Your Personal Effectiveness

The reason I research productivity is simple. I think that a productive life equals a happy life. Also, if you're more productive than average people, you'll advance faster in your career. You learn more. You do more. And eventually are rewarded more. And when I talk about productivity, I talk about being effective. Because productivity doesn't suggest that you get the right things done. It just means you get a lot of stuff done. But that's not what matters.

Effectiveness, however, refers to getting the right things done. And if you want to do your job well, earn money, live a meaningful life, or learn skills, that is what matters the most. Otherwise, you just run around in circles. You might appear busy, but you won't achieve anything meaningful.

In other words: It's easy to do useless work. Work that doesn't bring you closer to the outcomes you desire.

Results matter the most.

Practically, that means this: You might work for 50 hours a week, but if you don't experience any growth personally, emotionally, financially, you're not effective. People often ask me, "where do I begin?" To answer that question, I want to share one exercise that I teach in my productivity course, Procrastinate Zero. It's an exercise that I picked up from Peter Drucker's The Effective Executive. To me,

Drucker is the first and best thinker when it comes to effectiveness for knowledge workers.

Many of the books, articles, productivity tools, and productivity apps you see these days are all in a way influenced by Drucker, who essentially invented the term personal effectiveness. What you will find next is a simple exercise from The Effective Executive (which I modified slightly to make it easier) that you can apply to become more effective yourself.

Step 1: Know Thy Time

I often hear people saying: "I don't know what's wrong with me. I keep procrastinating."

My question is: "Do you know thy time?"

If you don't measure your time, it's tough to stop procrastination or improve your productivity. Because if you want to manage your time better, you have to know where it goes first. Your memory is not sufficient. If I asked you what you were doing exactly one week ago at this time, would you have an answer? There you go.

How do you know your time? Keep an activity log.

Before I even have a real session with clients, I often ask them to keep an activity log for two weeks. An activity log is exactly what you imagine — an hour by hour record of what you're doing throughout the day. The specific method you use for your activity log doesn't matter.

The only thing that matters is that you want to keep a record for at least two weeks. Preferably, you want a whole month of recorded activities. I just keep a pen and a notepad on my desk and every hour I write down the time and what I've done during the past hour. It's important to keep the notebook visible, so you don't forget.

Step 2: Identify The Non-Productive Work

This step is actually very simple. I just have one question for you: **"Go through all the recurring activities in your log one by one. What would happen if you would stop doing them?"**

If the answer is: "All hell breaks loose." Don't change anything. But if your answer is: "Nothing would happen." You've hit gold. We all do activities that have ZERO return. I call those activities time-wasters.

Step 3: Eliminate The Time-Wasters

Boom. That's it. Know where your time goes. Identify the critical tasks from the trivial tasks in your life. And cut the trivial, time-wasting, tasks.

"That simple?" Yes.

If you want to be a super effective person, you regularly keep a log. You don't have to keep a log for 365 days a year. Instead, do two stretches of two-three weeks a year. That's enough to keep track of your time and identify new time-wasters.

Also, the additional benefit of such a simple exercise is that it forces you to think about your daily routine. Often, we start time-wasting activities, and they become habits. And if you don't become aware of the pointless behavior, it's difficult to break those bad habits. I've found this exercise to be one of the most powerful things in productivity. Start now. Your activity log probably looks something like this:

- (insert time) — Read Darius Foroux' article about keeping a time-log and started my own time-log.
- (insert time) — Turned off my phone and got back to (whatever you were working on).
- (insert time) — Browsed the news, Facebook, Instagram. And watched YouTube videos. (Be honest with yourself. Shit happens).
- (insert time) — responded to emails.

Great. I'm happy to see that you started. Now keep going for another two weeks.

The Habits Of Unproductive People You Don't Want To Copy

The reason I study productivity is that I'm an unproductive person. I truly am. I sleep too much. I talk too much. I read too much. I listen to music all day. I watch movies. I buy gadgets that turn me into a zombie. If it weren't for my productivity system, I'd get nothing done. I wouldn't even write this article. But if you browse social media, all you see is super productive, healthy, and wealthy people. Is that really the case?

I don't know. I just know this: You can't be productive 24/7. And a big part of being productive is about getting rid of unproductive habits we all have. What follows is a list of ten unproductive habits that I learned to do less, or eliminate. Do you have a few of these habits? Don't worry; we're all unproductive at times. But if you have five or more, it might be time to change. One thing is sure: No one wants to be an unproductive person.

Working Too Much

Some days I can work 12 or 13 hours straight. I only take a break to exercise and eat. And I can keep that up for a few days. But after a few days, there always comes a crash. Big time. I struggle. I can't get stuff done. I don't even want to get stuff done. It's not good. So I learned to be more calculated with how much I work. Hemingway tried to stop at the height of his day. That's also my new goal. But that's hard because we always want things fast, fast, quick, quick, now, now. Just know yourself, your work, and your deadlines. Don't have a deadline? Take it easy because you need that juice for stressful times.

And most importantly: Have patience.

Worrying Too Much

What if I go broke? What if I lose my job? What if she doesn't love me? What if I get cancer? What if this plane crashes? What if I lose my sight? What if I...?

You got your head so far in the sand like an ostrich that you can't see how self-absorbed that way of thinking is. It's always about me, me, me. I know all about it. The above examples are all from my personal life. I used to be the king of the 'what if' game. But here's the thing:

YOU'RE NOT GOING TO DIE RIGHT THIS SECOND.

Get over yourself. Stop worrying. And do something useful. (I know, it's not that simple, but still: You can learn how to stop worrying.)

Being Stubborn

We deal with people all the time. Do you ever think: "Why should I listen to this guy?" Or: "What does she know?" I don't know. Maybe more than you do? We just don't know until we listen to others. But if you always think you're the best in the world, you never give people a chance. I think everyone is stubborn. Some are extreme, and some are just a little stubborn.

I must say, stubbornness is also a good trait. It's good to be deaf to critics and not care about what people think. But being stubborn in relationships is plain frustrating. That kind of stubbornness is not good. And it just so happens to be that life is based on relationships. And your career too. So when you refuse to work with others, you're sabotaging everyone else that's involved. Just remember that.

I try to remind myself often that stubbornness can be bad. But sometimes it's so bad I don't even listen to myself. But I keep trying.

Checking Things

What are you doing? "I was just checking Facebook." What are you "checking"? Email? TMZ? CNN? NBA? NFL? Instagram? Twitter? Snapchat?

Checking is not a useful thing. It might be a verb, but it's not a real action. When I started blogging, I always checked my stats for no reason. Then I thought: What's the outcome of checking?

Nothing.

You just consume information. I try to keep my "checking" at a minimum. That's why I deleted all news and social media apps on my phone. I don't even have email on my phone. Otherwise, I check it all the time. I don't want that. I only want to check my email when I have time to answer emails. Checking is a habit that you can never fully eliminate. I still follow the NBA because I like it. Pick only 1 or 2 "checking" vices you actually like. Eliminate the rest. You're not missing anything anyway.

Escaping Life

Until two years ago, every time I'd get stressed out, I said stuff like: "I need a drink." Or: "I have to go on a vacation." And when I had issues at work or in my relationship that became too much to handle, I preferred to pretend they didn't exist. Sometimes I would take some time to talk about it. But there are always deeper issues at play. Back then I didn't like my job, relationship, and the city I lived in. I basically didn't like my life.

Did I change it? Nope. I always tried to escape my issues. Escaping problems gives you some stamina to face your shitty life again. But you and I both know that problems never go away until you grab them by the root and extinguish them. I learned that the hard way. These days I deal with problems before they become big problems.

Saying Yes

Most people are afraid to say no. Maybe you don't want to let people down. Maybe you are uncomfortable with the word no. I don't know. Doesn't matter, really. What matters is this: If you keep saying yes, you're living someone else's life. Think about it. Deep down, we all know that it's true. We're not even in control of our own time. Want to be in full control of your life? Say no to a million things and yes to a few things that matter.

Not Writing Things Down

Yeah, yeah, you have the memory of an elephant. Or you're so smart that you remember everything, right?

WRONG.

Not writing down your thoughts, ideas, tasks, etc, is stupid. Why? Because you're wasting a lot of brain power when you rely on your memory. When you write everything down, you can use your brainpower for other things. Like solving problems. That's actually useful and advances your career.

If you journal, that's even better. But I've found that not everyone likes the idea of journaling. So let's just call it "writing things down."

What did you write down while you're reading this article?

Being Hard On Yourself

"I suck!" No, you don't.

"Why?" You got out of bed this morning, right?

"Yeah." Congratulations. You survived this hard thing called LIFE. Be proud of yourself. Everything you do after getting out of bed is a win.

Neglecting Your Personal Education

"Woohoo! I finished college. Goodbye lame old books!"

If that was you, no matter how long ago, you DO suck. Who learns one thing and stops forever? I don't even know why we have that idea planted in our brain. I always thought that learning stops when you get out of school. But the truth is: Your life stops

when learning stops. Invest in yourself. Learn something. Read books. Get courses. Watch videos. Do it from home or go places. It doesn't matter. Just learn new things. You'll be more productive and more excited about life.

Hating Rules

I saved the best for last. Most people hate rules, right? It starts when we're kids. "Why do I have to do this? Why do I have to do that?" Because it's better for you! That's why! (you weird kid) But when we're adults, we don't have to follow the rules (other than actual rules set by the government, but you get what I'm talking about.)

"Rules are dumb!"

That's what I always believed. I thought I was a maverick. But I was an idiot. Rules are actually THE BEST thing about life. Without rules, we would be hotdog eating pigs right now. And when it comes to productivity, the first rule is: Have rules. If you want to live without rules, go ahead. But life is not Fight Club. Rules actually help us to solve problems and get the most out of life.

Josh Weltman, an advertising creative director for 25+ years, and the co-producer of Mad Men, put it well in his book Seducing Strangers:

"Solving a problem requires a weird combination of freedom and constraint. Whenever I hear "Just have fun with it" or "Think outside the box," I know from experience that things are about to turn into a colossal waste of time."

Good news: You make up the rules.

For example, one of my personal rules is this: Never complain. Another one is: Read and exercise every day. And: Close the day every evening by setting your next day's priorities.

When you combine all your productivity rules, you have a system. Voila! And a system changes everything.

I rely on my system to work smarter, better, happier, and effectively. It took me years to figure out that a system is a good thing, and a few more years to create one, but it was worth it.

Because now, I get to be a productive person.

Not bad for an unproductive person, huh?

This 30-Minute Evening Ritual Will Help You To Kick Life In The Ass.

After a busy day, it's quite challenging to wind down and get ready for a good night's sleep. Too often I find myself working until late. And sometimes I might find myself reading or watching a TV show. And when you're ready to go to sleep, you can't. Your mind is buzzing with thoughts you don't want at that time of day. It's no secret that a lot of people have difficulties with sleeping. According to the National Sleep Foundation, 45% of Americans say that poor or insufficient sleep affected their daily activities at least once in the past seven days. Why's the evening so important? Well, you might have a perfect morning ritual, a fully planned calendar, and the intention to crush your day, but if you lack the energy, you're not doing anything productive.

During the past six months, I've experimented a lot with evening and morning rituals. What I've found is that a morning ritual is easy to implement in your life. But they're also easy to quit. When we wake up tired, we often fall back on our, not helpful, habits. End result? You lose, and life wins. You end up not focused, out of control, agitated, and just not happy overall. That's why I've created an evening ritual that helps me to get ready for some well-deserved rest. We all know it: Get 7–9 hours of sleep. But too often life gets in the way, and we don't follow common sense.

But with the following evening ritual, I've found a good way to bring more consistency in my evenings, and therefore, my life.

From minute 0 to minute 10: Close The Day

Every evening I take 10 minutes to journal about my day. In a few sentences, I write about what I've accomplished, what I've learned, and anything that's worth remembering.

That simple exercise helps me to:

1. Remember what I did (sounds stupid, but we forget most things we do).
2. Review my progress and see whether I'm doing all the things that I *should* be doing (like reading, working out, spending time with my family, writing, talking to people I work with).

I've learned this exercise from Jim Rohn. He says:

"At the end of each day, you should play back the tapes of your performance. The results should either applaud you or prod you."

It's simple: Close the day before you start a new day. Also, close every week before you start a new week. Similar for every month, and every year. Sounds simple, right? It's one of those "simple" ideas that have a huge impact on your life.

From minute 10 to minute 20: Review Tomorrow's Calendar

This is essential. When you wake up, you want to know exactly what your day is about. Do you have any important meetings or calls? Deadlines, maybe? What do you have to get done? When are you working out? Do you have any pressing items on your agenda? When are you dealing with them? This simple exercise takes away almost all stress and anxiety I have. Most anxiety comes from unsolved problems. And often, we worry about problems that are not real. But when you say to yourself: I'm going to work on problem X from 10 AM until 11 AM, you can relax.

Also, there's nothing you can do late in the evening. Just go to bed, already. Leave the problem solving for tomorrow when your brain is fresh.

From minute 20 to minute 25: Prepare your outfit

"Oh, you're so vain." No, I don't want to unnecessarily stress my brain. Look, your brain is a muscle. And after a certain amount of decisions, your brain runs out of juice. And that means the quality of your decisions will decrease. That's called Decision Fatigue. But I'm not worried about that in the evening because I'm headed to bed so my brain can recharge. A few extra decisions won't hurt. However, those few extra decisions will hurt your productivity if you think about your outfit in the morning.

So why not prepare your outfit so you don't have to use your precious brainpower in the morning?

From minute 25 till minute 30: Visualize

Because I've gone through my calendar earlier, I know what my day will look like. Next up: Visualize the next day in detail. Charles Duhigg talks about this exercise in his new book Smarter Faster Better. Duhigg writes about how the most productive people visualize their days with more specificity than the rest of us. I prefer to do this exercise in the evening because when I wake up in the morning, I still remember what I've visualized. The result is: NO MORE snoozing. You won't believe how much I would hit the snooze button in the past. In fact, I would snooze so often that the alarm on my phone would just give up. The hardcore snoozers know what I'm talking about. Hit snooze so often, and you win. The opposite is true. Snoozing is for losers.

But I'm not losing anymore because of this 30-minute evening ritual. As a result, I go to sleep without stress, and I wake up with focus: I exactly know what I have to do to turn the day into a success. And that's what I want to achieve with this ritual. 30 minutes of your evening sounds like a pretty good ROI if you want to improve your life. So give it a try tonight and find out for yourself. But don't be surprised if you wake up tomorrow morning ready to kick life in the ass.

Why Disconnecting From The Internet Improves Your Focus

Modern life is pretty good. You're always connected to the internet, inside your home, and outside of it. With your smartphone, you have the world at your fingertips. Sounds great, right? NOT. Most people don't use technology but are rather used BY technology. Apps, games, videos, articles, commercials, TV-shows, are all designed to keep your attention. So without you knowing it, you waste countless of hours every single week. Your attention is all over the place, but not at the right place.

"To be everywhere is to be nowhere."
— Seneca

Why do you think Netflix automatically starts the next episode in 3, 2, 1 seconds? When that happens, you think: "Screw it, let's watch another episode." The same goes for YouTube. Why do you think their suggestions are so good? They keep you locked in. And this applies to all content. There is ALWAYS a "next" video, episode, article, game, round, movie; you name it. Funnily enough, most people who read these type of articles know that a lack of focus is bad. And in recent years, a large number of research papers and books have appeared about the harmful effects of distractions.

Specifically, research shows that distractions are associated with more stress, and higher frustration, time pressure, and effort. Doing focused work is HARD. We're always distracted. And it's not your fault. Most technology taps into your lizard brain and locks you in — it turns you into a consumer. So don't even think about resisting the internet or technology. I bet you've tried it in the past. "I'm never going to browse mindlessly for hours." Yeah, right!

What will work? I've written about how I beat procrastination by creating a system. Well, one of the most critical parts of that system is this:

DISCONNECT FROM THE INTERNET.

And there's only one reason to do that: Too much of anything is a bad thing. Even good things.

- Too much exercise? You will get overtrained.

- Too much love? You will smother people.

- Too much work? You will burn out.

- Too much food? You will get fat.

- Too much water? You will die.

So why do you consume so much internet? I asked myself that question 2 years ago. I had no answer. So I thought; I do everything else in moderation, why not the internet?

Soon I found out that there's no moderation with internet usage. It's like an all-you-can-eat buffet. You're already full, but you still keep eating. And after you've stuffed yourself, the regret will eat you up alive. And that's the same with internet usage. It's so tempting and satisfying, and available EVERYWHERE. So you go all out with it. YouTube,

Whatsapp, Facebook, Snapchat, etc. I'm all about eliminating distracting stuff. However, I also don't want to live my life as a recluse. So I had to find a middle ground that worked. I've found that a simple tweak in my attitude towards the internet did the trick.

I went from "Always Connected" to "Always Disconnected."

In practice, it works like this:

- On my phone, wifi and mobile data are standard off. I only turn it on when I need it.

- On my laptop, I use an app called SelfControl during the times I work (try FocusMe for Windows). The app blocks distracting sites. The advantage is that my apps like Evernote, DayOne, Office 365 remain connected so I can save my work in the cloud.

"Always connected," isn't a good thing for your focus and productivity. It's the same as going to the gym. Or having dinner. Or having a romantic evening with your partner. You don't do those things for 24 hours a day.

You do them for thirty minutes, an hour, or a few hours. Too much of those things is simply not effective. Being disconnected from the internet has worked wonders for me. I don't feel the urge to check my smartphone, email, or the news 500 times a day anymore. And after a while, you feel like you're not missing out on anything. That brings a sense of calmness to your life.

I also get more out of my days; I achieved more things than ever, feel less distracted, and have more time to spend on the things that make me happy. At the end of the day, the internet is just a tool.

However, some of us think it's everything. But I'm pretty confident that, in years from now, I will not look back and regret that I didn't spend enough time on the internet. Can you imagine? You're on your deathbed, and you're saying this to your family: "I'm glad I watched so many FAIL compilations on YouTube." Nope. You'll probably look back and reflect on the time you spent with your family or friends. Or the memories you made when you were traveling. Or how much you enjoyed your work.

So cut the crap with the internet. It's not giving you anything but frustration. And after reading this article; disconnect.

You will get some withdrawal symptoms like grabbing your phone 100 times. Or hitting the F key on your keyboard (for Facebook) all the time. But I'll promise you this: Disconnecting will help you DO more. And that's what life is about.

The Single Biggest Reason Most People Procrastinate In Life

For most of my life, I've been a habitual procrastinator. When I had my first summer job at age 16, I did everything not to work. I had an inside sales job at a telecom company, and I had to sell mobile contracts to clients.

The company had software that would automatically call the next client when you finished a call. So you would be on the phone constantly — but I found a way around that process. After every call, you had to log your activity on the system. Things like "client is interested, but has to discuss it with her grandson."

Yes, I sold to a lot of elderly people (not proud of it). As a professional procrastinator, I took a lot of time to craft a lengthy summary of the call. When my manager asked me about my low number of calls per day, I told him, "If one of my teammates calls the client, they know she had to talk to her grandson. That's valuable information, right?"

I did everything to put off the next call. I also procrastinated during my years at university—pursuing a master's degree in marketing. I always waited until the last moment to finish an assignment or study for an exam.

I even procrastinated when I worked as a freelance marketing consultant after I graduated. "I'm doing research." This time, I told myself. I didn't understand why I always put off things to the last moment. I thought it was a part of my character.

And many of my friends were similar; they would say: "Who wants to work? Let's have some beer." This is what I believed: "Work is something you don't like to do — you just do it because you need money and status." Sadly, many of us believe that is the truth. Fortunately, my procrastination behavior changed this year. It wasn't some kind of magical productivity hack or software that turned me into a productivity machine. I'm more productive and focused than ever. And I'm more satisfied with my work than in the past.

Do you want to know the secret? I'm finally doing something that I love.

That's it. Work is not bad at all — I love to write, that's why I do it 7 days a week. I didn't like my previous jobs, businesses that I started, and I sure didn't like to study for classes I had zero interest in. Previously, I thought that you procrastinate because you have poor time management skills. That's why I've tried every productivity hack, system, or software, but they are all useless when you compare it to doing meaningful work. Do you want to get stuff done? Do stuff that matters.

Productivity hacks get a lot of attention. And very often, people present with time-management tips as a solution. In a way, time-management reminds me of speed reading. Many of us want to speed read to finish more books in less time. But why?

I enjoy reading—I don't want to spend less, but more time on reading. It seems like we want to skip the actual work and only focus on the outcome. It's like Ryan Holiday, author of

The Obstacle Is The Way, says in his article about speed reading: "If you find yourself wanting to speed up the reading process on a particular book, you may want to ask yourself, "Is this book any good?" Life is too short to read books you don't enjoy reading."

I think you can apply Ryan's quote to your life and career as well: *Life is too short to do work you don't enjoy.*

No matter how many productivity hacks you try, you won't produce more if you're not passionate about what you do. If you find yourself regularly procrastinating, you may want to ask yourself: *Am I passionate about my work?*

If the answer is no, you know what you have to do — find something that you are so passionate about that you don't want to procrastinate for one second. We all know that time is finite, so why not behave accordingly? If you know that you have limited time on this planet, why waste it?

"We all sorely complain of the shortness of time, and yet have much more than we know what to do with. Our lives are either spent in doing nothing at all, or in doing nothing to the purpose, or in doing nothing that we ought to do. We are always complaining that our days are few, and acting as though there would be no end of them."
– Lucius Annaeus Seneca

I'm a believer of 'do what you're passionate about', but I'm also a believer of 'do what you're good at.' The sweet-spot is right in the middle — a job that you love, and are also good at. Ramit Sethi, author of I Will Teach You To Be Rich, says that work and passion go both ways. He says that when we get really good at our job, we often become passionate about it.

I'm not saying that productivity tips are useless. In fact, I've written about productivity tips that improved my output. What I am saying is that the best solution for procrastination is doing meaningful work.

And procrastination can be a sign that you're doing something that's not meaningful. Don't let procrastination become a habit. After all, the worst procrastination is putting off your dreams and goals. If you're waiting for the right time, Benjamin Franklin says: "You may delay, but time will not." If you don't listen to me, listen to him.

This Ancient Habit Will Maximize Your Focus

Ever since I was little, I worried about many things. My favorite topics were money, health, and my future. What's your favorite topic to worry about? And don't tell me you never worry or fear nothing. Because if you have zero fear, that means you're a robot! Everyone spends time thinking about things that will never happen. Because that's what fear is. Michel de Montaigne, the 16th-century philosopher, said it best:

"My life has been full of terrible misfortunes most of which never happened."

We all know that fear is meant to save us from trouble. But in the modern world, that's simply not true anymore. These days, fear is only something that occupies your mind. Our thoughts are so cluttered with fear, worry, and stress, that we can't focus on our goals. In my personal experience, living a full life has nothing to do with the resources or opportunities you have.

It's about knowing what you want, and also knowing how you can get it. That's why you need to be focused every day. Without work, no goal will ever be achieved. That's why I want to share one ancient habit that stood the test of time. This habit has proved itself over and over again.

The Power Of Having A Mantra

I'm not a spiritual person. I believe in coincidence and luck. I also don't believe in some kind of spiritual energy that we can't see. I'm a pretty skeptical person. But I'm also a pragmatist. I believe in what works. That's why I never challenge religion or spirituality because it works for millions of people. In fact, I study religion, cultures, and different beliefs that people have.

And one thing that I've learned from religion is how useful a Mantra is. Most of us have heard about it, but few of us have one or, let alone, actively practice it. What is a Mantra, anyway? A good definition I found online is this:

"A "mantra" is a sacred utterance, a numinous sound, a syllable, word or phonemes, or group of words in Sanskrit believed by practitioners to have psychological and spiritual powers."

Mantras exist (in some shape or form) for centuries. You can find them in Hinduism, Buddhism, Taoism, and Christianity. I've learned that people from all over the world use a Mantra to overcome fear and improve their focus. It doesn't matter who came up with it first. What matters is that it works.

My favorite example of someone who applies it is Floyd Mayweather.

Yes. The boxer. Mayweather might be a controversial figure that people either love or hate. But he's also considered as the best boxer of all time. Not one of the best. Thé best. He has a record of 50–0. And he never even came close to losing. His recipe for success? A lot of talent, that's for sure. But, the man also has a crazy work ethic. And he's been training ever since he was a baby.

I've been following him for years. I don't care about his cars or money. I watch his training videos to see whether I can learn something that I can apply to my own life. A person with those kinds of results must do things right. You can't deny that. A few years ago, I noticed something that seemed like a promotion technique at first. Mayweather often repeated the same phrase:

"Hard work. Dedication."

It sounds like a lame company slogan. He says that while he works on the heavy bag, speedball, pads, and even while he's running. Constantly, he repeats the same words. Sometimes in a different order. And it wasn't until I learned about Mayweather's Mantra, that I started using my own. I always thought it was something that yoga hipsters use to become "Zen." Do you see me sitting on the floor with crossed legs and saying: "Hmmmn. Hmmmn. Hmmmmn"?

"Let's go."

That's my mantra. I've trained myself to say it every morning when I wake up. It really energizes me. I wake up and immediately say, "Let's go." I've experimented with different Mantras. In particular, ones that you repeat more often. But I've found that it's not my thing. I'm a pretty direct and no B.S. person. I prefer something short and powerful.

Not only do I say it when I wake up, I also say it before I start working. Or, when I want to start my workout. "Let's go." Give it a try. It works really well for me because it changes my state of mind to action. Especially when I feel afraid or powerless in life, I try to force a change in state. You know that platitude, "The only way out is through?" I believe that's true. And if you want to get through things, you need action.

After you start using your Mantra, you get into a worry-free zone.

This is one of the most effective things I've found in all of personal growth. I highly recommend a Mantra for everyone. All you need to do is pick a slogan that helps you to get focused, and that changes your state. Give it a try now.

"But I don't believe it!"

Pessimists say: "Just saying three words won't help you with real problems."

To those people I say: What will help? Drowning in your own misery? Being paralyzed? Never taking action? Complaining? Feeling bitter about life?

Never. We all know that life's too short to spend worrying about things that will never happen. And if something bad does happen to you, do something about it.

How To Focus Better: Manage Your Attention (not your time)

How many minutes of undisturbed work do you get done on an average day? 10, 20, maybe 50 minutes? If you think that sounds low, just examine your life. Most of us can't go undisturbed for more than 10 minutes. We're all so connected that it becomes impossible to find time to focus on yourself and your work.

Some of us get hundreds of notifications and messages per day. You find yourself answering a Whatsapp message here, an email there, talk to a friend, and then talk to a colleague on Slack. Most people's days consist of answering to notifications. In a way, you're held captive by others.

So no wonder that many of us ask: "How do I focus better?"

When new subscribers join my newsletter, I always ask them about their challenges. And the majority who answers, mentions something that's related to focus. In fact, when I did a survey on my newsletter last year, 28% said that their biggest challenge is related to focus and time management. Here are just two examples of what readers mentioned to me:

- "My number one challenge in life, and career, is trying to stay focused on my tasks. My mind always starts drifting to trivial things when I'm at work."

- "My biggest challenge is: how can we define what to really focus on?"

These questions have been on my mind in the past too. And you know what I found? Distractions are not some 21st-century first world problems. Distractions have always been a part of life. It has nothing to do with your smartphone or YouTube, online shopping, Instagram, or any other thing you want to blame for your lack of focus. It's human nature. We love to be busy. Socrates, one of the founders of Western Philosophy, warned us 2400 years ago:

"Beware the barrenness of a busy life."

Busyness is not a good thing. Because busyness and distractions go hand in hand. Want no distractions? Move to the woods. But that's not how life works. Plus, modern day life is too good. Seneca, one of the most famous Stoic philosophers, said this in Letters From A Stoic:

"There is never a time when new distraction will not show up."

There are always distractions. So you better train yourself to manage your attention. Not your time. Because that's the biggest mistake people make. We falsely believe that we can manage time. But time can't be managed. The only thing you control is your attention.

And remember: Focus determines the quality of your life. No focus means no control of your attention. And no control means frustration. We all know what frustration leads to.

Start managing your attention. Not your time.

Part II: Improving Productivity

"It's like a lot of things, said the smith. Do the least part of it wrong and ye'd just as well to do it all wrong."

- Cormac McCarthy

Smartphones Harm Your Productivity More Than You Think

Believe me, that thing you're using to read this article is not your friend. And even if you're reading this on your laptop or PC, there's one thing I want to ask you: How important is your device to you? I was shocked when I read a weird statistic a while back. An experiment, which was conducted by the universities of Würzburg and Nottingham Trent, revealed that 37.4% of the participants rated their phone as more or equally important in relation to their close friends.

Weirdoes.

Seriously, what's wrong with people? 29.4 percent of those weirdoes even said their smartphone was equally important, or more important, to them than their parents. Or is there something wrong with me? Am I just an old school person who likes to read books all day and only has a few close friends and family members that he actually values? Look, I'm not joking around.

Smartphones are dangerous. Not because they may cause stress, anxiety, and even depression, but because they change your behavior. It seems like we can't focus on one thing for more than 5 seconds. Why? Well, we can't because our smartphone is constantly going off. Not because people are calling you (it seems like people are afraid of calling these days, but that's another topic), but because you're constantly getting notifications about THINGS THAT DON'T MATTER.

Change Your Smartphone Behavior

The same study I mentioned above also found something else:

"Researchers asked participants to perform a concentration test under four different circumstances: with their smartphone in their pocket, at their desk, locked in a drawer and removed from the room completely."

The results are significant — test results were lowest when the smartphone was on the desk, but with every additional layer of distance between participants and their smartphones, test performance increased. Overall, test results were 26% higher when phones were removed from the room." Sure, it's just a study. And you don't have to believe everything you read. But this is something I can personally attest. For the past two years, I've significantly changed my smartphone behavior. Namely:

- I have turned off ALL my notifications except messages and calls

- I've removed myself from all Whatsapp groups except for one with my closest friends

- I've removed all news apps (if something important happens, you'll hear it from the people around you)

- I only consume music, paid journalism, articles from specific authors I follow, podcasts, YouTube videos (mostly to learn, but also for entertainment because I'm not a robot), books, and audiobooks on it

- For the rest, I use my phone to call, text, and to take notes, photos and videos

Also, I've stopped immediately responding to notifications. That doesn't mean I don't value other people who try to reach me. It means that I refuse to be a slave to my phone. I control my phone. For most of us, it's the other way around. In the past, Facebook, Instagram, Apple, Google, etc, all controlled my mind. Obviously, they still do because the only way to escape those idiots is to cut yourself off and run to the woods. That's not realistic.

I like my phone. But I don't need it.

The results have been great since I started using my smartphone in the above way. During the past two years, I got more things done than ever. And, I still have time to work out daily, hang out with my friends, have dinner with my family, and spend time with my lady friend. You and I both have the same 24 hours at our disposal. The difference maker is how you spend those 1440 minutes each day. To be honest, I think I still have much to improve about my effectiveness. No one reaches peak productivity. Nor is it important to be the most productive person in the world.

How you want to spend your time is your business. But please don't tell me you don't want to be 26% more productive by just changing one unimportant thing in your life: Your smartphone behavior. And if you wonder why not more people telling you to get rid of that thing, realize that they are trying to get to your wallet.

Also, social media people who claim that they run their business with their smartphone are doing the exact same thing. They need you to consume their content, on you guessed it, your smartphone.

Apple will also never tell us, "don't mind buying the new iPhone because it's going to destroy your productivity." Of course not, they try to tell you the opposite. And without a doubt, smartphones also improve productivity.

You probably found my articles on your phone. That's awesome. And, I also read a lot of articles and books on my phone. But you and I use the device to learn something, which is always a good thing.

People who make phones and apps are smarter than us. Their only goal is to get you hooked. I think it's good to realize that. That's why I often try to remind myself not to depend on smartphones too much because my attention matters more than productivity. It's time to reclaim your attention. And thereby, reclaim your life. It's worth it.

How Perfectionism Is Destroying Your Productivity

Do you always worry that you didn't do a good job? Do you always question your work and your actions? Are you afraid of admitting your mistakes? Does rejection make you feel like shit?

If so, you're in great danger. I'm not a perfectionist myself. At least, that's what I try to tell myself. I bet that you try to tell yourself that as well.

In fact, the people who don't admit it are the worst. But here's the thing: If you're a perfectionist, you're just a procrastinator with a mask. It's no different from someone who's lazy and does nothing at all.

Don't believe me? Let's take a look. A perfectionist...

- Always waits for the right moment.
- Never makes mistakes.
- Always needs more time.

But at the end of the day, life and work are about outcomes. Results matter. And if you're a perfectionist, you might get the outcomes *some* day. But the question is: When? And, at what cost? Research specifically shows that perfectionism is closely related to depression and low self-esteem.

"Perfectionists are their own devils." —*Jack Kirby*

Is the price of perfectionism really worth it? I've found that perfectionism is just another form of procrastination. When you constantly worry about making mistakes, doubt creeps in your mind. And that causes indecision. There are two types of perfectionists:

1. **The one that never starts.** You want to achieve something, but you immediately start doubting yourself. You think: "I don't think I can do it." So you never start.

2. **The one that starts but has too high standards.** You set a goal. You work hard (maybe too hard). But you've set your goals so high, that you're always failing yourself.

Both scenarios can cause the following: Anxiety, worry, depression, and Type A behavior. These are things that we rather avoid. Joachim Stöber and Jutta Joormann, who studied Worry, Procrastination, and Perfectionism, write:

"The combination of concern over mistakes and procrastination may be a crucial factor in the maintenance of worry. On the one hand, it may prolong existing threats because no steps are taken to cope. On the other hand, it may increase existing threats or even produce additional threats because initially solvable problems will pile up, thus creating an overload of problems that may finally be insoluble."

And that feeling of being helpless is the biggest pitfall for us. Because what do we do when we feel helpless? Exactly—we give up. Just look at the studies about Learned Helplessness. However, perfectionism is not always bad. In fact, some studies suggest perfectionism is related to greater achievement. But that's not the question here.

Of course, when you set higher goals and if you have higher standards; you achieve more. Without a doubt, perfectionistic tendencies can be a good thing. But as we all know, achieving goals is not the only thing in life. It's more about HOW we reach our goals and aspirations.

"How can we beat the nasty side of procrastination and perfectionism?"

So we've talked about how procrastination and perfectionism are related, and why it can be bad. But what's the solution? I've found an interesting study by Gordon L. Flett and his colleagues; they talk about the role of learned resourcefulness to perfectionism. They suggest that learned resourcefulness can play a mediator role. So I started looking into learned resourcefulness. And this is what I've found from an article by Michael Rosenbaum:

"Learned resourcefulness refers to the behavioral repertoire necessary for both regressive self-control and reformative self-control. This repertoire includes self-regulating one's emotional and cognitive responses during stressful situations, using problem-solving skills, and delaying immediate gratification for the sake of more meaningful rewards in the future."

Learned resourcefulness is the skill that you need to stop sabotaging yourself. Finding a balance.

Let's look at the opposite of a perfectionist: A slacker. If you're a slacker, you don't care about much. Good enough is your motto. And you have no ambition at all. An attitude like that doesn't bring you anywhere. The American novelist Cormac McCarthy put it best:

"It's like a lot of things, said the smith. Do the least part of it wrong and ye'd just as well to do it all wrong."

Slacking is an attitude of "I don't care." But if you want to make things happen in your life, you *have* to care. And what you want is to find a middle ground where your perfectionistic tendencies drive you, but you have the calm of a slacker, and you combine that with learned resourcefulness.

So that's why I found a balance between perfectionism and slacking. It looks like this:

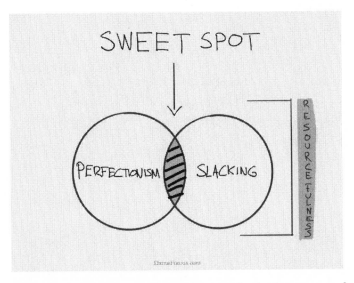

Do great work like a perfectionist, but don't give too much attention to your goals like a slacker. And finally, combine it with this:

- **Resourcefulness** — Goals can work well, but they can also be counterproductive. That's why you want to rely on systems. And when shit hits the fan; use your problem-solving skills to figure things out.

To me, that's the sweet spot: Instead of beating yourself up when you make a mistake or if you fail yourself, you just adjust or solve the problem.

- Avoid the perfectionist's favorite sentence: "OMG, this is the worst thing ever!"

- Also avoid the slacker's favorite sentence: "I don't care."

- But instead, you say: **"I've got this."**

So what's your current challenge? Actually, I don't even have to ask: You've got this.

How To Read 100 Books A Year

Does your reading list keep growing? Did you buy books that you've never read? It might be time to cross more books from your list this year than ever. If you're reading less than you want, you're not the only one. One year ago I looked at my Goodreads page and noticed that I had read only five books in 2014. That realization frustrated me.

I love books, but since I graduated college in 2011, I'd been reading fewer books every single year. My work and life got in the way of reading as much as I wanted. Why read 100 books in a year? You read because you want to learn from other people's experience. Otto von Bismarck put it best:

"Fools learn from experience. I prefer to learn from the experience of others."

If you want to get anywhere in this world, you need to educate yourself, and to educate yourself you need to read—a lot. Here's how to do it.

1. Buy In Bulk

It costs money to buy books, and it costs you time to read them — I'm assuming you have both if you're reading this. Everyone can make time. And if you don't have money, find a way to make or save money.

As Dutch Renaissance man Erasmus once said:

"When I have a little money, I buy books; and if I have any left, I buy food and clothes."

Be assured, the money and time you spend on books are worth it. I can't think of a better investment. Books are only a waste of money if you don't read them. If you want to read more, you have to buy more books. Some people don't get it. They spend $200 on new shoes, but they find it ridiculous to buy 20 books from Amazon.

The idea is simple: If you have more books in your house, you'll have more choices, and this will help you read more. Here's why: Most of the books you read are not planned in advance. You don't sit down in January and say: "The first week of June I'll read this book." You finish a book, look at your inventory, and decide what to read next. Don't overthink which book you should read next—you'll end up reading reviews for hours, which is a waste of time.

For example, most people who want to start with Stoicism ask me: "Which one should I read first—Seneca, Marcus Aurelius or Epictetus?"

Buy them all. Read them all.

Having an inventory of books keeps up the momentum. You also never have an excuse not to read.

2. A(always) B(e) R(eading)

You might have heard of the term 'ABC' from the play/movie Glengarry Glen Ross: Always Be Closing. Many salespeople and entrepreneurs live by that motto. I live by a different motto: Always Be Reading. I read a minimum of 1 hour per day on weekdays and even more during the weekend and holidays. Find a way to read around your schedule and your life situation. Don't make excuses like you're tired or too busy.

Always Be Reading means that you:

- Read on the train
- Read while you're breastfeeding your baby
- Read while you're eating
- Read at the doctor's office
- Read at work
- And most importantly — read while everyone else is wasting their time watching the news or checking Facebook for the 113th time that day.

If you do that, you'll read more than 100 books in a year. Here's how. Most people read 50 pages an hour. If you read 10 hours a week, you'll read 26,000 pages a year. Let's say the average book you read is 250 pages: In this scenario, you'll read 104 books in a year.

With that pace—even if you take a two-week break—you'll read at least 100 books in a year. That's a good return on your time investment. What's the ROI of reading the news? I don't know exactly, but it must be negative.

3. Read Relevant Books Only

Have you ever read a book that's supposedly amazing and you don't get it? I wouldn't go as far as saying that any book sucks because people spend a lot of time writing and editing a book. But not all books are for everyone. A book might be a best-seller, but maybe you can't stand the writing. Or maybe it's not the right time to read a book. In any case: If you can't flip through the pages, put the book away and pick up something you are so excited about that you tear up the pages.

Read books that are close to what's going on in your life. There's a book for everything you can think off. People are writing books for 2000 years, and there have been plenty of people in your shoes: struggling teen, aspiring artist, broke entrepreneur, new parent, etc. Don't waste your time reading about subjects you have zero interest in.

Instead, pick out the books that are related to your profession or hobby. Read books about people that you admire. Don't read a book just because it's a best-seller or a classic if it has no meaning to you.

4. Read Multiple Books Simultaneously

There are no rules to reading so you can do whatever you want. At times, I'm reading 5 books at once. I might read 50 pages of one book in the morning and then read another book in the afternoon. That's how I prefer it. Others like to read a book cover to cover and only then read something new. If you're reading something that's complicated, you might want to read something that's easier for the evenings.

I like to read biographies before I go to sleep because they are like stories. Fiction also works well in the evening. I don't want to read a book about investing in bed with a highlighter and a pen. If I do that, I will be awake until 3 AM because my mind is buzzing with the new things I'm learning.

5. Retain The Knowledge

Knowledge is only good if you use it. To retain knowledge, you need a system that helps you do that. This is how I do it:

- When you read a book, use a pen to make notes in the margins and highlight important text. If you're reading digitally, be aware of over-highlighting. Just because it's so easy you shouldn't highlight everything you find slightly interesting. Keep the highlighting for 'aha' things only.

- If you read something you want to definitely re-member, fold the top or bottom corner of the page. For digital readers: take a picture and store it in a notetaking app you prefer.

- When you finish the book, go back to the pages with the folds and skim your notes.

- Write down (use your notetaking software or physical notebook) in your own words what the book is about and what advice the author is giving.

- Copy the quotes that stand out the most to you.

The point is not to copy the book but to help you process the information so you can use it later.

Read as much as you possibly can — but never forget to apply what you've learned because that is what counts the most. You put in many hours to read books, make sure you get something out of it.

Take A Vacation: It Boosts Your Productivity And Reduces Stress

You recharge your phone when it runs out of juice. You refill your gas tank when you're running on empty. But sometimes, you forget to do the same for your most precious possession: Your body (and the brain that's inside of it).

Whether you love what you do, are in between jobs, or have a job you hate: You're working. 'Living' is also a job. A pretty tough one, actually. Just the act of getting up in the morning can be a daunting task. And I'm not even talking about all the responsibilities we have.

So, why do you make your life even more challenging by not taking a vacation to recharge? I'm not talking about your weekends that are packed with activities, or holidays where you work more than relax. No, that type of "free time" doesn't serve a purpose. I'm talking about resting with a very specific reason: To recharge your battery so you can keep working hard. To me, life is about working hard. Voltaire said it best:

"The further I advance in age, the more I find work necessary. It becomes in the long run the greatest of pleasures, and takes the place of the illusions of life."

Rest reduces stress. Improves creativity and productivity.

Scientific research shows that a vacation decreases perceived job stress and burnout. Now, that's a pretty solid benefit of taking a few days off. But there's more. As you may know, I'm always interested in productivity. In the case of resting or a vacation, my question is: Will I get more things done when I get back? The answer is yes, but there's one major thing to keep in mind. But let's back up a bit: What does it mean to get more done? Getting things done has nothing to do with time—if you work more hours, you don't necessarily get more done.

In fact, research shows that working more hours general means less productivity. Why? Well, we often waste time if we have more of it. It's simple: If I say to you, you have a year to write an article. What would you do? Procrastinate, right? But what if I tell you that you only have 2 hours? You immediately think, how can I write this article ASAP! So in a way, having more days off, and fewer days to work, forces you to be more effective with your time.

Research shows that a vacation in itself won't make you more productive, but when you have more days off, you have a strong desire to get more things done in less time. And that's a win-win situation for everybody: You, your business, or your job. You take off a few days, recharge, spend time with your family or friends, and when you come back, you're more productive.

Sounds great. But wait, there's a caveat.

When your vacation is stressful, the positive benefits go away. Have you ever watched National Lampoon's Vacation with Chevy Chase? That's how my family holidays were. Not good. So keep the stress at a minimum on your holiday.

Otherwise, you've wasted a perfect opportunity to relax and boost your overall productivity. Here are a few tips that might help.

1. If You're A Planner, PLAN

One of my friends loves to plan everything. He loves itineraries and minute by minute plans of the day when he is on vacation. I'm the opposite. When we went on a trip a few years back, he said, "I'm going to copy your style and just go with the flow." I said, "perfect." On the first morning, I slept until 10AM. It turned out he woke up early, got nervous because he didn't have a schedule, and spent the whole morning creating one. Don't try to be someone you're not. If you like to plan your holiday, just do it. But try to stay flexible: You're on holiday.

2. Make A Daily Movie

It's creative, and it's a great memory for later. Plus, focusing on the act of filming will force your attention on something specific. In that way, you will be more in the moment, and you'll worry less about stuff back home. Just don't film ALL day. Otherwise, you won't be present at all. All you need is a smartphone.

Just film stuff with your phone and edit it right on your phone. If you're more into video, bring a proper camera and a laptop.

3. Read A LOT

Bill Gates is famous for his voracious reading habit. He is

also known for his 'Think Week' where does nothing else but read and think. Recently, he published an article with 5 books that he's reading this summer. Take a look if you're looking for some inspiration. I like to read for hours on my holidays. Reading slows down time, makes you think, and is good for your brain.

4. Get Bored

One of my favorite strategies for finding new ideas is to get bored out of my mind. It sounds easier than it is because of distractions. In the past, I would do everything NOT to get bored: Watch TV, go out, browse Facebook, etc. But did you know that you can use boredom to your advantage? Instead of giving into distractions, just give into the boredom and see where it leads your mind to. In fact, one of my favorite artists of all time, Andy Warhol, embraced boredom. You can tell by the boring films he made or the references he made in The Philosophy Of Andy Warhol about getting bored.

Whenever I hit a creative wall, I just do nothing. Literally, nothing. Try it sometime. It's a great strategy; maybe you come up with the next best thing in your industry.

It's never a good time to take a break.

- "I just need to finish this project."
- "My boss will never accept it."
- "People will think I'm lazy."
- "I don't have time."
- "Money never sleeps."

Yeah, yeah, I've been there too. But what would you rather: Continue to work without resting and burn out? Or take some rest before you're tired? Yup, life is long—so play the long game.

On that note, I might not be tired yet, but it's time for me to take a break. So I will see you again when I come back on August 1 with a new article.

Until then—take it easy, because I definitely will.

P.s. For years I couldn't afford to go on a holiday. If you're in the same position, have a staycation. The above tips still apply.

Eliminate Mindless Browsing

We all have days we feel unproductive or that we did not do anything. When you feel you are not productive, the chances are that it is because interruptions and multitasking drain your energy.

When you juggle multiple things simultaneously, like; sending an email, text a friend and checking your Facebook while you are in a meeting, you engage in context switching. In a research done by Gloria Mark of the University of California, Irvine, it showed that it takes an average of 25 minutes to return to the original task after an interruption. Since we are interrupted more than once, this adds up quickly, and before you know it, you feel like you have done nothing that day.

Clifford Nass, a sociologist from Stanford University, has researched the impact of multitasking and found that people who engage in multitasking are "suckers for irrelevancy." We engage in multitasking because we are distracted by notifications, which are addictive.

We cannot control ourselves; we must look at the notification to see who or what wants our attention. Every time a notification pops up on our screen, we get a rush that releases dopamine.

Dopamine is one of the body's happy chemicals; it controls the "pleasure" systems of the brain and makes you feel joy. This joyous feeling is addictive and makes us seek out behaviors that stimulate dopamine. You can think about food, sex, drugs and the notifications you receive on your screen.

While dopamine may cause a rush, it also exhausts us. That is why you still feel tired at the end of the day while you have not been productive. This is a harmful process, and we need to stop this pattern.

The Fix: Eliminate Browsing

Being productive can be as simple as taking control over your day. What harms your productivity the most is *browsing*. It absolutely kills it. We've all experienced a distortion in time when we are browsing. "What?! I just did NOTHING for 2 hours." Yes, we even do this at work. Take control of your attention and time. The point is; do *something that's worth your time*. Be conscious about your time. And spend so it improves the quality of your life.

20 Things That Will Make You More Productive Than Ever

The last three years have been huge for me. I've got more things done than ever, moved countries, bought an apartment and a small office building, spent loads of time with my family and friends, kept a healthy lifestyle, and exercised at least 4 times a week. Many variables determine your overall productivity. Tools, apps, or hacks, don't work if you lack the right mindset because productivity is a way of living. It's about achieving maximum output, getting shit done, and not wasting time. I think that output and happiness go hand in hand. To me, doing nothing equals misery. I want to share 20 things I've done in the past three years that have made me more productive than ever (in no particular order).

1. **Always Cut To The Chase**
    With everything in life, there's a bunch of crap, and there's stuff that matters. Chit chat, small talk, delaying, waiting around, not speaking up, is all useless. If you want to get shit done, you have to jump straight into the action.

2. **Record All Your Thoughts And Ideas**
    Similar to computers, we have a Random Access Memory (RAM). Your human RAM stores relevant short-term information. But your RAM capacity is limited. When it's full, older information that you have stored will be deleted to make room for new information. You want to write down your

thoughts to unload your RAM, which gives you more brainpower. Even if you never take a look at that note again, it's still worth it.

3. **Say No**
   When it comes to work, I say no to everything that doesn't support my goals and values. We live in an abundant world — there are always enough opportunities. In my personal life, I say no to everything that doesn't thrill me. When I think 'meh' about something, I always say NO. That eliminates wasting time on shit that I'm not excited about.

4. **Take A 5 Minute Break Every 30 To 45 Minutes**
   You can stretch your back, walk around, drink some water. But more importantly, you take your nose out of your work. When you come back to your desk, you might have new ideas. Or, you might think: "WHAT AM I DOING?" And stop it before you waste all your time.

5. **Eliminate Everything That Distracts You**
   Willpower is overrated. If something distracts you, eliminate it. One of my friends has a news addiction. I suggested to get rid of his tv, delete his news apps, and block the news sites on his laptop. Two weeks later he told me that he's finally starting a business. Don't think you're immune to your distractions. Remove them.

6. **Keep Away Clutter**
   A cluttered life means a cluttered brain. And with a cluttered brain, you can't get stuff done. I prefer a

simple work and living environment. A desk, a laptop, and a notebook. Keep it simple. You don't need any fluff.

7. **Focus On 1 Thing Some Days**
   If you have recurring tasks, try to do as much of the same thing on one day. I write 2–3 blog posts on 1 day, the other days of the week I use for my other projects and businesses. On my writing days, I turn off my phone and just write. Nothing else gets in the way.

8. **Stop Consuming So Much Information**
   You don't need to read 5000 articles on productivity. If you find useful information, try it. Don't search for more. More is not always better. You can only process so much of it. Stop consuming, start creating.

9. **Create Routines**
   Decisions fatigue your brain. And routines eliminate decisions. Which ultimately means more brainpower. Routines are not OCD — they are efficient. Use them.

10. **Don't Multitask**
    When you juggle multiple things simultaneously, like; sending an email, texting a friend and checking your Facebook while you are in a meeting, you engage in context switching. In a research done by Gloria Mark of the University of California, Irvine, it showed that it takes an average of 25 minutes to return to the original task after an interruption.

That's a waste of useful time.

11. **Check Email Twice A Day**

    Every time you check your email, you get a rush of dopamine. I get it — checking email feels nice, and most of us are addicted. While dopamine may cause a rush, it also exhausts you. That is why you still feel tired at the end of the day while you have not been productive. To minimize that, turn off notifications, and check your email only twice a day on set times.

12. **No Smartphone During The First Hour Of Your Day**

    A smartphone's primary function is to interrupt you. But don't let other people or apps interrupt you during the first hour of your day. Take that first hour to think about the day ahead of you, read a book, enjoy your breakfast, coffee or tea.

13. **Plan The Next Day**

    Every night before I go to bed, I take 5 minutes to set my priorities (usually 3–4) for the next day. That makes me more focused when I wake up. I find that I waste time if I don't do this practice. It's cool to 'go with the flow.' The only problem is: I don't want to be a dog that mindlessly chases cars.

14. **Keep 'Thinking' To A Minimum**

    When people say: "I'm thinking." They mean worrying by thinking. Don't think too much. Just DO, and see what happens. If you like what you're seeing, continue. If not, do something else.

15. **Exercise**

    A few things are vital in life: Food, water, shelter, relationships, and exercise. Without this stuff you can't function properly. Scientific research shows that regular exercise can make you happier, smarter, and more energetic.

16. **Laugh A Little**

    Laughing reduces stress. And if you want to keep up your productivity, you don't want stress. So move the corners of your mouth upward as much as you can.

17. **Don't Go To Meetings**

    This is a tough one for people who work for corporations. Some companies have a 'Meeting' culture. People organize meetings just to look important or procrastinate real work. For goodness sake, PLEASE STOP.

18. **Is That Really Necessary?**

    Ask yourself that question as often as you can. You will find that your answer is often: Nope. So why do unnecessary things?

19. **If You're Having A Shitty Day, Press Reset**

    You might screw, maybe someone gets angry with you—shit happens. Don't get down about it. Take some time alone, meditate, listen to music, or go for a walk. Try to get back on track — don't let your day go to waste

20. **Do The Work**

> Yes, talking about work is easier than doing it. Everyone can do it. But you're not everyone, right? You're a productivity beast. So act like one.

Without these 20 things, I wouldn't be productive at all. You may have noticed that I don't get into details, like which tools and apps I use.

I don't think that stuff matters. It's about creating a productivity mindset and environment that lets you thrive.

I only care about getting things done in a fun and not stressful way. That makes doing work way more fun and rewarding.

Here's Why Time Off Work Actually IMPROVES Your Work and Life

What do you do when you feel tired or overwhelmed? Do you power through? Or do you take some time off? In the past, I thought that you should always power through — no matter what. Now, I still think that way when it comes to life in general. You can't quit taking care of yourself and your family. A sense of responsibility is one of the most powerful motivators in life. But I'm not talking about a lack of motivation here. I'm talking about taking time off work. But there's still a massive taboo on taking time off. Some people think it's for losers. Others think it's about escaping your work.

After all, "If you love your work and life, why do you even need a break?" Good point, smart ass. Here's why time off actually IMPROVES your work and life.

Leonard Mlodinow, a physicist, who also co-authored two books with Stephen Hawking, recently shared scientific research in his book Elastic about taking time off. He demonstrates that taking time off work improves our well-being:

"Though some may consider "doing nothing" unproductive, a lack of downtime is bad for our well-being, because idle time allows our default network to make sense of what we've recently experienced or learned."

People who never take time off to do nothing are short-term focused. "I want to reach my goals! NOW!" But as always, short-term thinking harms your long-term development and growth. What happens when you power through work and burn yourself out? In most instances, your results suffer, and you become less productive. In some cases, you even become depressed — which will set you back even longer.

Prevent Rather Than Cure

It's one of the biggest clichés in the book. But how often do we really prevent things? Instead, we put our head down and, "deal with it later." Bad strategy. Instead, it's much better to prevent burn-out or a decrease in your overall work performance. Dale Carnegie, a self-help pioneer, and author of How to Stop Worrying and Start Living, said it best:

"So, to prevent fatigue and worry, the first rule is: Rest often. Rest before you get tired."

So take time off work strategically throughout the year. That's what I just did too, and I experienced 5 benefits as a consequence:

1. You Can Check Whether You Did The Right Things

At work, I know two modes:

1.   Execution
2.   Thinking

When you are in execution mode, you can work for hours, days or months in a row. In fact, I know people who've been in execution mode for years. They never took time off to reflect or think about their work. Result? A midlife crisis. Or, young folks who experience a quarter-life crisis. That's what you get when you put your head down and execute without thinking. You might get results. But are those results what you WANT?

When you take time off work, you have more inner-conversations. But when you execute, you don't. That's one of the most important benefits of doing nothing. Sure, you might fall behind on work. But who cares? Would you rather go through your career with tunnel vision? I need at least ten days off to reflect seriously. For the first five days, I'm still somewhere between execution and thinking mode. It's hard to switch to thinking and doing nothing if you're used to doing work. But I always learn new things about myself after a more extended break. I tend to read a lot. Over the past two weeks, I've read five books. But I didn't write at all. Also, I journaled very little.

Just some reading, watching movies, documentaries, hanging out with friends, talking, daydreaming. That kind of stuff. Neither does it cost much. But the return is enormous.

Now, I feel better, have more energy, and I'm excited to get back to work. That's also the next lesson I learned.

2. You Get To Process Your Ideas

Your brain does a lot of things you're not aware of. One thing that happens unconsciously is the processing of ideas by our brain. We've all had ideas that never materialized, right? How many people have you met who claimed to have had the idea for Facebook, Instagram, or any other type of new thing? I once met a guy who claimed to have come up with the idea of making e-bikes. Did he do something with it? No. He now buys garbage on Alibaba and sells it to businesses, door-to-door. We all have ideas. Not only business ideas.

- "I want to redecorate the house."
- "I want to drive from NYC to LA."
- "I want to write a book."

All those ideas are great. But what are you going to do with them? I'm not even talking about execution. All ideas require processing. Are the ideas any good? Do I really want to do those things? Again, that's a thinking process. When you go from idea to execution, without processing, you often waste your time in hindsight.

Of course, you can never entirely prevent that. But by taking the time to process your ideas, you can prevent your future self a lot of pain, worry, and even money.

3. You Can Consume More Art

What is art? Anything that makes you think. A good song, movie, painting, book, poem, article, picture, sculpture, you name it. Anything can be art. There's no authority that declares what art is and what is not. I get a lot of my inspiration from art. I can't imagine what life would be without it. Well, there is art on that too. Just read Fahrenheit 451 or watch the movie Equilibrium. The best thing about art is that it improves your mood. And when you're in a good mood, you're happier.

Just don't consume useless junk. Start with the classics. Listen to Bob Dylan, Marvin Gaye, Whitney Houston. Watch movies by Alfred Hitchcock, Francis Ford Coppola. Read Ernest Hemingway, Harper Lee, Ralph Ellison. Go to the British Museum. Study Andy Warhol. Like millions of other people, you'll be inspired by their work. And that will enrich your life.

4. You Can Focus On Other Important Things (that are not work related)

"Can you tell me more about yourself?"

What do you think of when I ask you that question? Most of us start by saying something like, "I'm an accountant at company X." Modern day life almost forces you to identify yourself with work. But you are not your job. You are your family, friends, hobby's, passion, and then finally, you also have a job. And yes, work is important. But so are the other things.

So never neglect the other important things in your life. Cultivate the relationships you have with your family and close friends. Do things together. Go on a family holiday. Go mountain biking with your friends. Show some initiative. If no one in your family or group of friends takes action, why aren't YOU? By investing time in your relationships, you form group memories. That will only strengthen your relationships. But also focus on yourself. What are your hobbies? What's something you want to learn more about? What did you dream of doing? Do those things.

5. Resting Gets Boring. Quick.

There's a reason humans work. We're built to make things. I believe that the purpose of life is to be useful. Making yourself useful ultimately leads to a meaningful life that satisfies all your human needs. That's why too much rest will make us restless. My mother always told me that too much of a good thing becomes a bad thing. She told me that when I wanted to hang out with my friends all the time and when I had my first girlfriend.

It's true. Too much rest, like work, is not good. Our bodies and minds are made to use. Hence, the final lesson I learned from doing nothing is this: After rest comes work.

And what comes after work? If you answered "more work," you didn't get the point. You probably need some rest.

Time Blocking: Improve Your Focus And Get More Meaningful Work Done

Do you have a list of priorities or goals that you want to achieve this year? And do you struggle with allocating time to them? I'm no different. Life can be messy. Most of us juggle a lot of different things at the same time. Even though the simple solution is to stop juggling, it's not always realistic. Or even needed. What if you could do more things without losing your time? It's possible. But you must work in an organized way.

Enter: Time Blocking, a simple productivity exercise that many people use. It's not fancy or revolutionary. The only thing you need is a calendar, which is something everyone with a smartphone and computer has. Time Blocking is simply using your calendar to block time for your most important priorities. During that time, you only work on that one thing. And, you let your calendar lead the way. That way, you don't have to think, "What should I do next?" But Time Blocking is more than just a productivity tool. It's about self-awareness.

The road to high productivity starts with awareness.

For instance, one of my priorities this year is to write a book on pragmatic thinking. However, there's a problem: I haven't been writing.

How did I come to this conclusion? I simply looked at my list of priorities for 2017, and then I looked at my calendar. I hadn't scheduled any time for writing in a while. Now, you might think, "do you really have to look at your calendar to realize that?" Yes, I do. I'm not some kind of supercomputer that remembers everything. I'm a regular human being. I think of something to do, start working on it, life gets in the way, and then I FORGET about it. It happens to all of us. We need self-awareness and tools that keep us in check. And that's why I like Time Blocking.

Some people love Time Blocking. Some people hate it.

Computer science professor and author of Deep Work, Cal Newport, also uses time blocking. He says:

"I take time blocking seriously, dedicating ten to twenty minutes every evening to building my schedule for the next day. During this planning process I consult my task lists and calendars, as well as my weekly and quarterly planning notes. My goal is to make sure progress is being made on the right things at the right pace for the relevant deadlines."

The last sentence is exactly why I schedule everything I want to do. *Working* is not the same thing as *making progress*. And Time Blocking helps me to improve my focus so I can get *meaningful* things done. Things that have an actual impact on my life.

I know there are a lot of successful people who work with empty calendars. I've read the articles. They simply work two, three or four hours per day. And to be honest, that sounds very attractive to me too. However, one must look at his/her own life situation. What are you trying to achieve?

And more importantly: What resources do you have? Often, people who don't have a lot of money, *do* have a lot of time. So why not use it wisely? Either way, I think that planning serves a purpose.

I plan my days and weeks in advance because I want to make sure I'm working on the RIGHT things. Too often, I get lost in completing daily tasks. Think about it this way. I'm pretty organized already. And I only work on one big thing per area of my life. But there are many different areas of my life: My family business, my blog, podcast, online courses, relationship, friends, investments, etc. It might sound like I'm doing many different things. But it depends on how you look at it. Everything I do leads to one thing: Living a meaningful and independent life.

But let's not get philosophical here. If you're lacking focus, not making progress, and want to work in a more organized way, give time blocking a try. Here are some things I've learned that may help:

- Take 10 minutes every evening and plan your next day. Rearrange blocks if you must create time for other important things.

- Use recurring blocks for recurring tasks. For instance, I've scheduled two hours to write my new book every Tuesday and Thursday.

- Don't over-schedule. Realistically, you can't be productive 10 hours straight. Give yourself some time between tasks.

- And always schedule more time than you think

you need.

"Wow, that sounds like too much planning to me."

No problem. Plan less. There's always a counter-movement for everything. People who do the exact opposite and advocate an anti-productivity lifestyle. You know, folks who claim they have empty calendars don't care about anything in life. People who pretend they are always "enjoying" themselves. They like to go with the flow and daydream.

You know what that reminds me of? Those kids in school who always said, "Ah dude, I didn't have time to study for this class," but always ended up getting straight A's.

People just want to make you believe they don't work hard. It's a facade. And when they do well in life, it seems like it came easy.

As far as I know, achieving meaningful things is hard. I don't think there's anything cool about pretending it's easy. Nor do I believe that it's cool to work yourself to death.

I often think of this question: Are you an amateur or a pro?

It's Steven Pressfield's famous analogy, from his book The War Of Art, for getting work done.

The amateur only works when inspiration strikes. The pro sits down every day and puts in steady work. The key is steady. Not irregular or extreme.

I Stopped Working Out Daily. Here's What Happened.

For the past three years, I've been setting a yearly focus for my life. In 2014, I wanted to work abroad and travel as much as I could. In 2015, I wanted to read more than 100 books in a year. And in 2016, I wanted to work out every day of the year. I've done those things. I love setting a yearly focus because it gives you a clear idea of what you want to do with your time. You'll be surprised what you can do in a year if you put your mind to it.

This year, my focus is to write more books (even though it's not going great, I'm still working on that). But at the same time, I also don't want to stop reading and working out. However, that's sometimes more complicated than it sounds. In January of this year, I got the flu. And when I came back to our family business, I underestimated how much work I had to catch up with. I also wanted to keep creating new content for my blog and online courses.

I thought to myself: "I can't do everything, so I'm going to cut back on daily exercise."

BIG MISTAKE

Here's what happened.

- Instead of daily exercise, I went to the gym 2–3 times a week. And I ran once a week. (this was by the end of January)

- For the first few weeks, nothing was wrong, and I felt good. I was also productive.

- But by the end of February, that changed. I started feeling tired by the end of the day. Something that never happens to me.

- I also started writing less. I had a big buffer of articles, so I did post 2 articles a week.

- By March, I was at a productivity low. Fortunately, I always stick to my productivity system. I managed to get the minimum amount of work that's necessary done. But I stopped creating.

- I started watching Netflix in the evening. I even watched an episode of a TV show called 12 Monkeys. It was complete shit. I much more prefer to read a book before bedtime.

- So I got frustrated that I wasted my time.

- And when I'm frustrated, I start journaling and reflecting more.

- I looked at my habits. And I noticed I felt tired and got less work done.

- Why? The answer was: EXERCISE.

- Actually, a lack of it.

- **By April, I shifted my focus again: Get back in shape.**

So that's what I'm doing now. And if you want to get in shape too, it's important to understand what you're aiming for. For instance, I'm 6"3 and 181 pounds. But that doesn't mean anything.

Most common measures like the BMI are pretty useless because they don't say anything about your strength. To be honest, I don't care about measures or even my exact fat percentage. Instead, I look at my fitness and how it impacts my daily life. When I'm in good shape, I can:

- Run 5K at a fast pace without stopping for rest.
- Deadlift, squat, and bench press my body weight at least 8 times.
- And do at least 15 pull-ups.

What's that based on? My body and experience. In fitness, there's no general rule. You must find your own goal. To me, a person should be able to at least lift or push the same amount as their body weight. That helps you to function properly in daily life. When you're in good shape, you'll have more energy and focus.

Want to find your fitness goal?

Read books about fitness and health, watch YouTube videos, talk to experts, and then create a program that's for you—not a 21-year-old bodybuilder. Also, you don't have to lift weights. Find something you enjoy and challenges you physically at the same time. The cold reality is that if you don't use your strength and stamina, you lose it. But that doesn't mean you should neglect it. The same analogy that Zig Ziglar once used to stress the importance of motivation applies here:

"People often say that motivation doesn't last. Well, neither does bathing — that's why we recommend it daily."

So if you're not working out every day, you're not doing yourself a favor. The quality of life decreases when you stop working out. And stop looking for silver bullets to feel better. I know, it's not advice most of us like to hear. Exercising is hard. But that's the whole point!

The easiest solution for a good life is right at your disposal: Your body.

Are you neglecting it or strengthening it?

If You Want To Be More Productive, Research Shows You Need A Break

Do you spend the majority of your day at your desk? And do find it difficult to concentrate throughout the day? There's a simple solution to improve your productivity and focus.

"How can I get more stuff done without being distracted?"

That's a question I often get. It's human nature: We always want to improve output. For machines, it's straightforward: You improve speed. Machines get faster and better every day. But what about your personal productivity? I've read dozens of books on productivity. I've read countless articles on time-management.

And I've tested different methods to boost my productivity. The idea is simple: I want to get more done in the same amount of time. I'm not looking for shortcuts or hacks, so I have to do less work. I don't mind working. What I *don't* like is the feeling of wasting time on stuff that is meaningless. Sometimes I start by watching one YouTube video, and BOOM, 2 hours have gone by. And then I get frustrated with YouTube. But that doesn't make sense. It's like getting angry with alcohol after you've spent a night boozing.

It's not the alcohol, IT'S YOU. You just couldn't have *one* drink, or watch just *one* video. Couldn't you?

I've found a way to eliminate that frustration with the distractions of work (not boozing), which makes it a lot more fun to work and less stressful.

The solution is simple: Take a 5-minute break after every 30 minutes of work.

It's also called the Pomodoro technique. The reason this method works is also simple: Evolutionary biology. The human brain can't focus on a single task for long periods. Our brains are meant to ensure our survival.

To protect us from looming threats the brain is in a constant state of alertness. So focusing on one thing for a long time is hard for your brain. Research by Alejandro Lleras, from the University of Illinois, showed that deactivating and reactivating work allows us to stay focused.

When you are completing long tasks, such as studying for exams, making presentations or writing reports, it's best to take short, and planned breaks. Taking breaks will also increase the quality of your work. When you take a break, you force yourself to take a few seconds to reevaluate. Sometimes you find that you have to adjust your work to increase the quality.In contrast, when you work on a task, without a break, it's easy to lose focus and get lost in the work.

That's why the 5-minute breaks are equally important as the 30 minutes of work. Take your breaks seriously — see them as a reward.

Use your break to walk a bit, do some stretches, grab a cup of coffee or do something that relaxes you. Feel pleased with the work you have done. I've been working in 30-minute intervals for over a year. I've never got so much work done. I also find it more fun and less stressful to work. I've experimented with different time intervals (25, 30, and 40 minutes), breaks, and 45 minutes is pretty much the maximum.

Some research shows that it's counterproductive to focus for longer periods of time. So you can experiment with how long you prefer to work before you take a break. If you want to try this method, here are a few other things that can help:

- Use an app to set the 30-minute interval. I use Tomighty.

- Assign just one task to every 30-minute interval.

- Don't skip your breaks.

- Don't check your email during your break.

- Take a 15-minute break after 4 intervals.

- Don't accept interruptions or false emergencies when you're in a 30-minute stretch.

- Set a daily goal. For example; doing 10 x 30-minute intervals results in 300 minutes of productive work.

With all the noise, it's easy to forget the importance of taking breaks. You don't need to read another article about productivity. Instead, take a break.Sometimes we get lost in the lists and productivity hacks. The truth is that no matter what you do to improve your productivity—you still have to do the work. So you might as well get those 5-minute breaks to recharge.

Part III: Achieving More

"A man who chases two rabbits catches neither."

- Chinese proverb

Don't Know What You Want? Improve These 7 Universal Skills

What does success look like? What do you want from life? What career do you want? Most of us answer "I don't know." And you know what? There's nothing wrong with that. And yet, we think it's the worst thing in the world if you don't know what you want to do in life. We say: "OMG! I don't know what I want!" And then we have a full-on panic attack. Be honest — it happens to all of us.

Especially, when you see that your old college friend just got married. Or that your co-worker, who started at the same time as you, just got promoted. It's at those moments of weakness when we shine a spotlight on our own uncertainty about life. One of the biggest thinking errors that I've made was that I thought I needed to know what I *exactly* wanted to do with my life. The truth is that no one knows what they truly want.

Accept The Uncertainty

You could get killed by a cow tomorrow (really happened). You could lose half of your money on the stock market. Your property could go up in flames. I don't have to tell you all those things. But we must realize that we don't have the answers to most things in life.

Will you stay healthy? Will the stock market crash? Will your business continue to prosper?

NO ONE KNOWS!

That's the beauty of life. Eleanor Roosevelt said it best:

"If life were predictable it would cease to be life, and be without flavor."

Some people ask me, "Why do you read so many books? There's no way you can apply everything you learn." They are right. I cannot. Why do I still read about all kinds of different topics? There *might* come a time in my life where I will need one particular piece of knowledge. And that one time I need it *might* just change the whole outcome of my life. I'll give you an example. In 2015, after my friends and mentors told me I should share my ideas about productivity, life, and business with others, I seriously started thinking about doing it.

But there are many ways you can share your knowledge with others. You can give training to groups and host seminars. You can coach people individually. You can create videos for YouTube. You can give talks at conferences. The possibilities are endless.

But because I've always had an interest in writing and had read so much about it in the past, I realized that I should start with written ideas. That was the easiest way for me to get started. I had also learned all about creating websites in the past. So it was very easy for me to get started with all of this. In fact, I created a website in a day.

And I started writing every day for a month. The result? A book and a bunch of articles.

Know Your Direction. Not Your Destination.

When I read about writing and building websites years ago, I didn't know I would use that knowledge to build my own blog. To be honest, I didn't know what I wanted. I only knew what direction I wanted to go in. I knew I wanted to make a contribution and do work that I enjoyed. So it's not important to know exactly what you want to do with your life. People change. Economies change. So, it's not even realistic to boldly claim "I know what I want!" The only thing every person needs is a sense of direction. A vision of where you'd like to go.

Look, you don't need to know your exact destination. You often read about people who say they always knew what they wanted. But that's just a small portion of the population. I've personally never met someone like that. Most of us don't have that conviction from day one. It grows over time. If you can't decide what direction you want to go in life, that's automatically your #1 goal in life — to figure out where you want to go.

That's what Jay Abraham also recommends in Getting Everything You Can Out of All You've Got (which is one of my favorite business books of all time):

"Your first priority is to identify what you want and then make sure you take the path that's going to give you that. There's nothing sadder than to see someone get to be seventy-five or eighty years old and look back regrettably because they pursued the wrong target."

You see that he doesn't say you should know exactly what you want? That would not be realistic. Instead, we need to know where we're roughly going. I know, it remains intangible. But that's the only helpful answer that I've found in life.

Work On Universal Skills

While you're figuring everything out, don't waste your time watching hours of TV, drinking booze, or eating junk food. Spend your time usefully. Learn skills you can always rely on. Need some inspiration?

Here are a few skills that I'm constantly working on:

1. **Self-Discipline:** Get better at ignoring the negative voice in your head. Get out of your bed. Go to the gym. Don't listen to "I don't want to."

2. **Personal Effectiveness:** Learn how to maximize the results you can get during the 16–18 hours you're awake. Get more done — effectively.

3. **Communication:** We think we're all master communicators. But the truth is that we suck. Communication is both art and science. And our ability to work with others depends on it.

4. **Negotiation:** You negotiate all the time. With your spouse, kids, parents, teachers, friends, co-workers, managers, etc. Learn to get the best deal for all parties.

5. **Persuasion:** Learn how to get what you want in an ethical way.

6. **Physical Strength & Stamina:** Getting stronger is a skill. Pull your own weight. It's something every human should be able to do.

7. **Flexibility:** Sitting all day long behind your computer or in your car turns you into a stiff being. Learn how to stretch your hips, lower back, hamstrings, and calves — the most common weak points of desk workers.

That's enough to keep you busy for a lifetime if you want to do it well. Pick a skill that excites you. Get better at it. Then, pick another. And keep on repeating that process.

Soon enough, you'll know what you want. And if you don't, it's not the end of the world. There's still plenty to learn.

Leave The Office On Time and Don't Take Your Work Home

These two lessons are true for every person who wants a long, happy, and satisfying career. But it's very hard to put that advice into practice. It took me the first six years of my career to figure that out. And I still have to remind myself that life is bigger than work.

Almost everywhere that I've worked in the past, there was a *"perception is reality"* culture. That means looks are more important than reality. In other words: The person who's in the office the longest appears to be the hardest worker. Now, that may be true. But that's not what matters. We all know that the only thing that counts is results. However, we collectively insist on looking at vanity factors like participation in meetings, hours spent at the office, and how fast people respond to emails. It's pathetic.

At our family business, we encourage everyone to leave when they are done for the day. We've learned that focusing on priorities is a much better metric than only looking at the hours someone works. And still, people find it uncomfortable to say, "I've finished my top priorities, I'm going home." I get it. When you work in a group, you don't want to make others feel bad or that things are unfair.

But think about why you're working in the first place. You're there to contribute. To your own company, or the company you work for.

Working Too Long Is Unproductive

Now, I'm sure people love to be in your presence for 10 hours a day, but that doesn't mean you have to stick around so long that you become unproductive. Because that's one of the main reasons we've stopped working standard 9 or 10 hour days. It's useless. There's a large body of research that proves working long hours is counterproductive.

Working too much and the stress that goes along with it can lead to depression, sleep problems, impaired memory, and even heart disease. You get the idea. That's why my first rule of work is this:

Leave On Time

The other day I was talking to my mentor about how great it is to love your job. He said: "I've never had a job in my life that I didn't love. It's one of the most gratifying things in life." But like my mother always says, "too much of a *good* thing becomes *bad*." I believe that's the same with work. Now, I'm not talking about intensity.

Don't get me wrong; I work my ass off. Always have done. But just don't go on for too long. The art of working hard is knowing when to quit. But like my mentor told me, that's very hard: "My biggest problem was that I worked too much. I left the house at 7 AM and came back at 11 PM. That's too much."

You must protect yourself against too much work.

And it's straightforward. Just leave the office on time. Whether you love your job or not — it doesn't matter. When it's time to go home, GO! No one needs you to be at the office 24/7. Only your ego does.

Honestly, the office will be here tomorrow. Your co-workers will still be alive. Your company will not go bust. Work is about achieving results. If you can't do that in 6–8 hours a day, you're not effective. So instead of working overtime, read a book on personal effectiveness or get productivity training.

Leave Your Work At Work

But don't just go home and bring your work with you. That defeats the whole purpose. No one thinks it's cool when you're closing deals on the phone at dinner. You're also not doing yourself a service by continually thinking about work when you're at home.

Relax a bit. Play some Call of Duty. Cook dinner for your spouse. Take the kids for a walk. Whatever. Look, living a happy life is very simple. It's all within our control. We can decide what makes us happy. I have printed this Marcus Aurelius quote on my journal to remind me of that:

"Very little is needed to make a happy life; it is all within yourself, in your way of thinking."

We all know that money, success, fame, or recognition, by themselves, don't make us happy. And yet, we work too much to obtain those things that don't even make us happy in the first place. So why do we keep working too much that it hurts us?

It could be our ego. Maybe we just can't help ourselves. It's different for every person. Personally, I don't care about the reason. All I know is that too much work has a negative impact on the quality of your life and work.

What matters is that we protect ourselves from our own stupidity. We're just like kids. We need rules to live happily and safely.

That's why the first rule of work is that we leave the office on time. The second rule is that we don't take our work home.

And the third rule? Let's not worry about that for now. We'll get to that another time. It's time for me to go home.

Consistency Is Key: Improve By 0.1% Every Day

Do you ever worry about things you don't control? If you do, join the club. It happens to all of us. But worrying is a waste of time and energy. Imagine the following situation: You make a mistake at work that upsets a client. Maybe you send someone a wrong email. Maybe you forget to solve a problem. It doesn't matter what it is. Imagine that something goes seriously wrong at work.

What do you do when you find out? Do you stress out? Feel uncomfortable? Blame yourself? Blame others? Think it's the end of your career? When things go wrong, we become our own worst enemy because we focus on things we don't control. It's one thing to read about these things. It's another thing to actually put it in practice.

Because when shit hits the fan it's natural to panic. Instead of *thinking*, take a step back, and focus on what lies within your control. What do you control? Essentially, we only control our own actions and mindset.

We determine our:

- Desire
- Attitude
- Judgments
- Determination

That's about it. Anything else, we have no control over. So it makes no sense to worry about things that are not on that list. That's a Stoic philosophy exercise. Something that exists for centuries.

And the best thing is that you can immediately apply this to your life. Next time you catch yourself worrying about a situation, focus on the things you control. What counts is that we do the right thing because that is all we can do. We don't control outcomes. Do you see?

1. Made a mistake? Correct it.
2. Something goes wrong? Find a solution.

Also, never be surprised when bad things happen. But rather *expect* them to happen. In that way, you will never be caught off guard. Similarly, when you're struck with bad luck, don't complain and say stuff like, "why me!?" Instead, accept it, and then focus your energy on finding a solution. Always keep a positive mindset.

Why this exercise improves productivity.

I'm often asked, "what does philosophy have to do with productivity?" Well, if you want to be productive, the most important thing is **consistency**.

Productivity is not about eureka moments, your big break, pulling off all-nighters, or drinking Red Bull all day.

If you want to achieve things in your life, it's about aiming for daily progress.

You want to exercise, read, work, learn, study, every single day.

Inconsistency is the enemy of results.

And that's why I practice Stoic and Pragmatism philosophy to improve my mental toughness. It's also a big part of my personal productivity system, Procrastinate Zero.

I don't want ups and downs because that hurts productivity.

Instead, I want to progress 0.1% every day of the year. And that's a very realistic goal.

Try it and maybe it will change your life too.

Who Says You Have To Get Out Of Your Comfort Zone?

I love my comfort zone. To me, that's where the real magic happens. In my comfort zone, I have my family, friends, work, music, books, movies, bike, gym, park; you name it. Everything I love. And from that place of safety, I'm more open to trying new things and take risks. I've never believed the idea of that stupid little drawing. You know what I'm talking about, right?

- "Your comfort zone." A little circle.
- "Where the magic happens." A big circle that stands for the promise of success.

As if "magic" only happens when you step outside your comfort zone; that's ridiculous. And while we're at it; why pretend as if your comfort zone is bad? It's this pathetic little circle displayed against the bigger "magical" circle. Sure, I'm all about pushing yourself, trying new things, moving forward, growing, etc. But in contrast to many popular self-help people, I don't believe the comfort zone is a bad thing. Call me a pessimist. Call me a stoic. But more than anything, I'm merely a practical person. And practically speaking, you don't even want to make a huge leap outside your comfort zone. In fact, I believe in the slow road to "magic."

Where's The Magic People Talk About?

I've found that I do my best work when I don't worry about money, finding new friends, getting familiar with a new environment, and anything else that is related to always moving around. But don't get me wrong. I'm not saying I prefer to stay put. Stagnation is a death sentence for me.

I believe that there are different phases of life. Sometimes, you take it easy, work on your skills, your character—you invest in yourself. And sometimes, you just go out there and take a chance. Life's too short to be a wimp. But those two things are interconnected. If you don't work on yourself, and if you lack self-confidence, you will never take a risk. For years I wanted to do what I'm doing now.

But instead of jumping out of my comfort zone (which was scary), I slowly took on new and bigger challenges. First, I got two degrees in business. Then, I started a business together with my father. That was in 2010. And after two years of working on that business for six or seven days a week, I started doing freelance marketing work. Again, after a few years of freelancing and starting (and failing) other businesses on my own, I took a job at a research advisory firm because I wanted to know how it is to work for a major corporation.

And after doing that for a year and a half, I finally decided to write and talk about productivity, career, and entrepreneurship on the internet.

By then, I'd been doing the things I write about for more than 10 years. And yet, I don't have all the answers—I just share the stuff I've learned. So it would be ridiculous if I would join people who scream: "If you want to be successful, all you have to do is step outside your comfort zone. NOW!"

Well, have you ever stepped outside your comfort zone? Even just a little bit counts. And what did you find? A leprechaun with a bag of money?

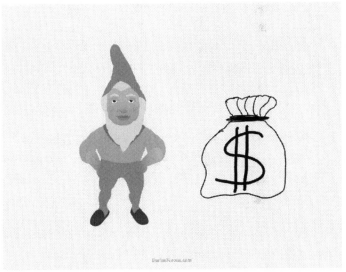

Not going to happen.

That comfort zone shit is just a story. It might motivate some people, but you don't have to believe it if you don't want to. It's just like when people claim you have to wake up early if you want to be successful. Says who? I believe this: If you step outside your comfort zone, there's only more work waiting for you. It's not fancy at all. There's no magic involved. Just blood, sweat, and tears.

Work Your Way Up From A Place Of Comfort

I think that most people who read these type of articles want to achieve something. Maybe you want to quit your job, start a business, grow your business, become an artist, publish a book, whatever. And you probably also know that it's not easy. So why do you make things even harder for yourself by doing shit that makes you very uncomfortable? Instead, start from the very bottom. Build a strong foundation. Get comfortable before you do scary stuff.

"How does that foundation look like?"

If you want to live stress-free, you need enough money in your savings account, so you can live and eat for six months in case things go south—see it as a fail-safe system. Again, that's my practical mind speaking for me. Make some calculations and figure your what that number is for you. And don't even think about taking a risk before you have that money on your savings account.

Also, build a skill set that's worth something. One of the reasons I don't care about money is because I trust my ability to find work. Even when I go broke tomorrow, I'll find a way to get work the next day. I've invested years and hundreds of thousands of dollars in my education. The question is: What's your skill? How can you add value to the world?

What problems can you solve? Other things that complete your foundation:

1. **Family.** If you don't have a family, create one.
2. **Friends.** You can't be friends with everyone. Stick to a few people who also stick to you.
3. **Yourself.** Consciously improve your body and mind. Go to bed a little stronger and wiser every night.

Lastly, don't try to be something you're not. If you're an introvert, don't pretend that you can work in a boiler room. If you're an extrovert, don't pretend you can work in solitude. Stay close to yourself—there's no point in pushing yourself so badly that your life becomes miserable. In the end, we all need comfort: It's one of our basic needs as human beings. But we also need growth. So whatever you do, don't stay in your comfort zone for too long.

Try to keep moving forward every day: Even if it's just a tiny step. No magic. Just effort.

If You Can Believe It, You Can Achieve It

I know what you're thinking. "This guy probably read a motivational quote on social media, and now he's telling us that nothing is impossible. Yeah right." I think the world has no shortage of motivational articles, books, videos, or Facebook posts. You don't need a bigger dose of #mondaymotivation. You know why? That type of motivation is not practical. It doesn't do anything. It's not useful. It's the same as drinking Red Bull. It fades quickly. Belief, on the other hand, is a tool that's extremely useful. And it's underutilized by many. The problem is that most of us lack belief. And when I talk about belief, I talk about it from a practical point of view.

I'm not talking about hope or faith. I don't believe that you can "hope" for the best, sit back and wait until good things happen to you. Hope is not a strategy for life. I prefer to look at facts and make conclusions like a pragmatist. Like it or not, but everything that's floating in that head of yours is there because you believe it.

- "Life sucks."
- "I'm not good at my job."
- "I can never find my dream job."
- "No one loves me."
- "I will never become successful."

See? It's all there because you believe those things. William James, one of the primary figures associated with pragmatism, put it best:

"Belief will help create the fact."

Belief is a practical instrument that you can use to shape reality.

Have you ever considered that you decide what you believe? Not your friends, colleagues, family, or even the media. You observe things, and then decide what you believe. That's why belief creates facts. No, life is not an R. Kelly song. You can't fly, no matter how hard you believe it.

A pragmatist always keeps it real.

- You will never become a respectable leader **without putting in the work**.
- Your life will never change **unless you take action**.

But that's not the point. You know this. There's no outcome without action. It comes down to one thing: Do you believe that you can, or can't live the life you want? It's as simple as that. But it's something that you truly have to believe. It's one thing to say that you believe something. It's a whole different thing to actually believe.

Let me highlight that by sharing a personal story. For most of my life, I lived in fear. It all started at school. People told me:

"If you don't get good grades, you will not be accepted to a good university, and without a good degree, you will never get a job, and you will become a bum who dies alone."

After hearing that, my seventeen-year-old brain went into a full-fledged panic mode. I started believing that stupid story.

Who wants to become a bum and die alone?

That's a metaphor for not believing in yourself. Because somehow, that's always the alternative. If you do something that's uncommon, or maybe a little risky, the common argument is that you become homeless. I meet a lot of people who say they've made important life decisions based on fear.

- Do you hate your job, but are you afraid to look for something else because you might lose your house?

- Do you want to leave your spouse, but are you afraid you'll die alone?

- Do you study yourself to death because you're afraid of what your parents will say when you quit?

- Do you never expose your work to the world because you're afraid people will throw rocks at you because you suck?

Will that really happen? Or is that just your mind acting up? Probably the latter. I always wanted to become a writer. Back in school, I wrote poems for my girlfriend. It was kind of pathetic, but hey, she enjoyed my weird poems. But all jokes aside, I loved to read and enjoyed putting my thoughts on paper. But no, every adult in my life was trying to scare me to death. "You can't make a living as a writer." They were probably right. It's not easy to make a living by writing. So what? Everything that's worth it is hard. I didn't realize that back then. So I gave up my goal. I decided to pick the safe road and pursue a degree in business. I don't regret that decision because I've learned many useful things. But the whole experience turned me into a fearful creature. Because after that whole scarefest in school, I eventually stopped believing in myself. I stopped writing and reading. And that's a pure waste of time that I could've used for practicing my skills.

You can achieve anything (as long as you believe in it).

What's something you once believed in but stopped believing because of fear? I think we've all been there. If you're not careful, you'll always stay there.

For me, it wasn't until two or three years ago that I figured out belief is an instrument that can help you to achieve your goals. Somehow I started reading about pragmatism (which is a way of thinking). And it completely changed my own way of thinking. I realized that not believing in yourself is useless. So I decided to believe that I could live the life I wanted. Granted, I'm not fully paying the bills by writing yet. I run a business and do consulting. But I do make some money with my blog. And that's pretty good to know for the seventeen-year-old version of me. Believing in yourself is very simple. You can do it too. Just understand that belief is an instrument. That idea is not new or anything. It's been around for hundreds of years. People just have different names for it.

I don't care how you call it. But guess what happened since I've been using belief as an instrument? Most things I believed are facts now. And the other stuff I believe will one day become a fact.

How am I so certain?

Because my mind can conceive it. And if your mind can conceive it, you can achieve it That's not a motivational quote. That's a fact.

Do you believe it?

Don't Compete. Create!

If you think that you have to *compete* for better jobs or more market share, you're as wrong as I was.

The idea of competition is engraved in our minds. We believe that we have to compete for the same jobs with others. If someone has a job, that means you can't have the same job. And if a company has a certain market share, that means you have to compete with that company to "win" a piece of their share. At least, that's what conventional advice says. It's also what I learned in business school. My entire education was based on *competing* with other businesses. And almost every business book that I've read, also assumes that business is competition.

They couldn't be more wrong. When you assume that you have to compete with other businesses or people for money, jobs or attention, you're engaged in limited thinking. Instead, we must adopt an abundance mindset. Wallace D. Wattles, one of the first famed personal development authors, said it best:

"You get rid of the thought of competition. You are to create, not to compete for what is already created. You do not have to take anything away from any one."

The biggest mistake that conventional business thinkers make is that they believe supply is limited. But that's not always the case. But even if it was the case, it's harmful to adopt that mindset. I think that most people, entrepreneurs and those who are employed, are afraid that someone else beats them to "it." Right? We fear that we lose our clients, business, contracts, attention—and that we lose everything we worked so hard for as a result.

But that's exactly the problem. Fear begets fear. When you're afraid that you won't be able to grow, what will happen? Exactly, you won't grow!

Life Is Abundant

A quick look at history shows that mankind always kept moving forward. Sure, we've had times of war and economic downfall, but we always recovered and grew. So when you're expecting that the world economy will not grow, you're actually betting against mankind! I don't believe that. Humans always find a way to survive and prosper. That's simply what we do.

You must believe that we live in an abundant world. There is enough opportunity and riches for everyone. So, never allow yourself to think that you won't make it. What is that good for?

If You Can't Find The Right Career, Create One

You know, life is not easy. And it's also not easy to find a career that truly satisfies you, both mentally and financially. I know that millions of people face that challenge. But I also know that many of these people limit themselves by thinking that they can't create a career. Similar to how I think entrepreneurs and companies should create market share, I also believe that individual people should create a career.

I recently met a "Chief Happiness Officer" at a non-tech company—which is pretty unusual. I did some research, and it appears that Ronald McDonald was the first who had the CHO title in 2003. After that, tech companies started adopting the title. It's very simple. A CHO is responsible for the wellness and happiness of employees. I also read that Tony Hsieh, CEO of Zappos, is a big advocate of employee happiness. But here's the thing: Traditional companies think it's bullshit. Initially, the company I mentioned before shared that thought. And naturally, they didn't have a CHO position. She told me she had to *create* the position. In the past, leaders believed that the only reason people will work for you is because of the salary. The more money you offer, the better the people you attract.

That might be true for some. But more money is not always better. Many people care more about having fun at work, feeling appreciated, and being happy. And that's what the CHO does successfully.

Here's the thing: It doesn't matter what others think. If you believe in something and if you can *create* value, go for it. There are always people who say things like:

- No one needs this
- Your work is garbage
- You're wasting your time

Don't listen to the naysayers. Let them drown in their own limiting beliefs. Instead, do this:

Create. Create. Create.

There's enough opportunity for everyone in the world. The problem is that most people don't *use* the opportunities.

If you want to have a specific career, go out there and create it. The same is true for your business. And don't focus on limited resources, naysayers, or any other reason you should *not* do it.

Adopt an abundance mindset. Before you know it, you'll have so much opportunity that you don't know what to do with it.

In The Netherlands, we call that a "luxury problem."

Believe me; it's the only problem that you want to have.

All Strength Comes From Repetition

The biggest mistake you can make is to ignore the basics of your profession. This is true no matter what you do, where you live, or who you are. When you ignore the foundation of what makes you a good person, athlete, friend, entrepreneur, student, etc., you will never be consistent. That's the biggest lessons I've learned from studying athletes. People who play professional sports are under constant pressure to perform.

Take Daniel Cormier, the current UFC Light Heavyweight Champion, and former Olympic wrestler. The 38-year-old champion has an impressive career until now. He won multiple gold medals as a wrestler. And in MMA, he has won 20 of his 22 fights in total. He's considered as one of the best. On top of that, he's also a combat sports analyst and co-host of UFC Tonight on Fox Sports. The man is highly active. What is his key to success, according to himself? Focusing on the basics. He says:

"You don't get to the highest levels of the sport without having the basics in order."

That's not only true for sports; it's also true for everything else in life. Writing, speaking, selling, leading, you name it. Without having the basics in order, you'll never achieve your full potential.

Repeat The Basics

And there's only one way to improve the basics, by repetition. You get stronger by lifting weights, rep after rep. You build stamina by performing anaerobic exercise. We all know that. But how about your mind? How do you become mentally stronger? And why does it even matter? The answer is simple: Everything starts with the mind.

Steven Pressfield, the author of The War of Art, said it best:

"Long-term, we must begin to build our internal strengths. It isn't just skills like computer technology. It's the old-fashioned basics of self-reliance, self-motivation, self-reinforcement, self-discipline, self-command."

But my challenge was always: How do you do that? I know how to get physically stronger. But I never knew how I could get mentally stronger. And whenever people told me "it's all about life experience" I always thought there was a better way. Let's be honest, who wants to wait until they are 70 to get mentally strong?

Some things can be done faster, especially if you keep repeating the basics. Because that's when we screw up most of the time. We think we know everything.

Stay A Beginner

How often do you think to yourself, *"I already know that"*?

If you're like most of us, quite often. One thing we have to remind ourselves is that the people who think they know everything are the biggest losers in life. I meet people all the time who think they know everything. And I don't even mention people on the internet. A lot of commenters always want to show how smart they are and that this is "so obvious." Well, that's not how the greatest people in the world approach things. Muhammad Ali once said that:

"It's the repetition of affirmations that leads to belief. And once that belief becomes a deep conviction, things begin to happen." When you repeat the basics, you don't only become great; you will *stay* great. It's a challenge that all high performers face. I repeat the basics of many things in my life: Fitness, philosophy, kindness, business, writing. For example, I re-read my favorite books on Stoicism every month to exercise my mind.

I regularly grab The Elements Of Style by Strunk & White to repeat the basics of simple and effective writing. If I don't repeat these things, I simply forget about my philosophy for life or how to write good articles. That's how our brain works. Without repetition, we forget things easily. I always look at myself as a beginner. That's one of the first (and most important) lessons I learned from my mentor. He's now in his seventies and still considers himself as a student of life. I have the same approach to business.

I always go back to the question of, *"what is the purpose of a business?"* I can tell you that if you answer, "to make money," you need to repeat the basics.

It's very simple: Figure out what the basics are in your field. And repeat them. Keep it simple. There's no bigger waste of time than repeating bad, wrong, or negative things. That's the only thing you should be mindful of. Don't take advice from people who haven't successfully done something themselves.

Be Great. Stay Great.

Look, you can be very smart, driven, humble, etc., but if you don't *stay* that way — what's it all worth? How often do you see people become successful only to squander their success? How many one-hit wonders have you seen?

Exactly. Only the great ones are here to stay.

And if you want to stay here too, you must never underestimate the power of repetition. Never think you've made it or that you're smart enough. Because that mindset is what *keeps* you great.

How I Measure My Life

You can easily measure a business by looking at the numbers. Turnover, profit, costs, employee churn, etc. But how do you measure your life? There are no universal metrics to assess your life. So it's up to every person to create their own way to measure where they are in life. Some do that by looking at how much they earn compared to their peers. Some look at how far they climbed the corporate ladder. Others measure themselves by how they look. I have studied how the most successful thinkers of our time measure their lives. The answer is surprising. You rarely hear that successful people measure their life by the size of their bank account or any other conventional measure. Instead, people who're considered successful in the eye of society often look at these 3 factors:

1. Energy
2. Work
3. Relationships

I've experimented with improving all the three above things. What I've found is that they are all closely related. When I have high energy, I'm in a good mood, and when I'm in a good mood, I do better work. And when I do better work, I feel satisfied with my life so I can give more to the people in my life. And that improves my relationships. And what's the secret to a good life? Good relationships.

Clayton M. Christensen, a Harvard Business School professor, and author of How Will You Measure Your Life? writes:

"The single most important factor in our long-term happiness is the relationships we have with our family and close friends."

When it comes to relationships, quality matters more than quantity. Though it's easy to pick on people who are influenced by social media, I still think it's worth saying: No one cares about how many followers or online friends you have. Real relationships take a long time to grow. And they are also unconditional. Most relationships are not real. We only love someone until they, for example, change their views or gain a few pounds. Or we only invite friends to our birthdays as long as they go out with you and drink beer.

These types of conditional relationships are worthless. Real friendship and love are stronger than that. You support the people you love no matter what. That makes life rich.

1. Measuring Energy

Measuring your energy is easy. All you have to do is look at how you feel physically. I recently wrote about that specifically. What matters is that you find ways to increase your energy. You can start by asking yourself one question: What small thing can I do today that has a significant impact on my energy?

Here's something that is true for everyone:

1. **Exercise every day** — I lift weights four times a week, do two interval runs, and make sure I walk at least 30 minutes at a fast pace on the days I don't work out.

2. **Eat well** — I don't follow a specific diet. I eat meat, bread, pasta, and a bunch of other things that are supposed to be bad for you. But I feel great. I just don't eat processed stuff, and I eat very little sugar (I like chocolate). I also don't consume more calories than I burn.

That's one part of the equation. When I do those two things every day, I feel great. And my energy is also high. As soon as I stop working out or start eating unhealthy, I feel down. That's how I know this works.

You can easily improve your energy by exercising more and eating well.

2. Measuring Work

When it comes to work, I don't look at income, status, or other generic measures. Instead, I look at how much I can still learn. In other words: Have you reached your full learning potential?

Why do I look at learning and not income? Because it matters more.

Christensen puts it well in How Will You Measure Your Life?:

"In order to really find happiness, you need to continue looking for opportunities that you believe are meaningful, in which you will be able to learn new things, to succeed, and be given more and more responsibility to shoulder."

Career and life success is directly related to how much you learn. And more importantly: How much you *keep* learning. Education never ends. Also, income is directly related to your learning development. The more you learn, the more you earn. It's true. Of course, there are limits to this statement. And knowledge must always be put into practice. We've all heard about the smart people who've wasted their potential. To be successful, you must always act on what you know. Without action, knowledge is useless. But generally speaking, the more knowledge you have (from experience or studying), the more you can contribute to your company, colleagues, clients, etc. And contribution translates to income.

3. Measuring Relationships

What you'll find is that the more you contribute to other people's lives, the better your relationships will be as a result. And that final ingredient completes the circle of life. When you measure your relationships, only stick to yourself. Avoid the biggest mistake most of us make: We look at what others do for us. Otherwise, you risk that you start keeping score.

"How people treat you is their karma; how you react is yours." As the late Wayne Dyer said.

Instead of looking at how others treat you, measure how much time and energy *you* put into your relationships. That's the only thing you can control.

My experience is that when you make time for the people that matter to you, the relationships improve. And if they do not, the relationship was probably not meant to be. We simply have to move on.

The real lesson here is that we always must focus on what we can control.

Our energy, our effort at work, and what we put into our relationships — these are all things we control. It's one of the main lessons philosophers from all over the world and from all ages tell us.

Look at your life. Make a quick assessment of how you feel. All you have to do now is to improve it.

Why You Should Live Like You're Immortal

It seems like all my peers have this idea that being young is an excuse for not living a satisfying life. But millennials are not the only group of people who hide behind excuses. We all do. I get it. Taking on responsibilities in life is scary. It's way cooler to have toast with avocado.

But you know what's also cool?

- Building a meaningful career that you're proud of.
- Contributing to other people's lives.
- Creating a product or service that is useful.
- Investing your money for your retirement.

"Yeah, but I'm still young."

"There's always tomorrow!"

C'mon. Stop hiding! What are you waiting for? To everyone out there that doesn't feel fulfilled, I have one idea that I want to share:

Start living like you're immortal.

Yes, I know it sounds weird. So give me two minutes to explain. Conventional wisdom says that life is not forever, right?

- "Life is short!"
- "YOLO!"

- "Live now!"

And I agree with that as well. But when you live your life according to that philosophy, it doesn't make sense to do anything that takes a long time to pay off. If you think that life is short, why on earth would you do hard things? It doesn't make sense. From that perspective, it's better to spend your money, go out every week, drink as much as you can, and live large.

Ask yourself: "What does all that lead to?"

It doesn't take a scientist to answer that question. The answer is, "nothing." Now, there's also another perspective on living: That you're here forever. Think about it. How different would you live if I told you that you're never going to die?

When I look at myself, I used to live as if I were mortal. I'd spend my money on clothes, gadgets, holidays. But I also seemed to be in a hurry. I wanted to achieve a lot of things in my life. And preferably, very fast. I also pursued many things at the same time. Just like a dog. Chasing every shiny thing out there. Or even chasing my own random ideas.

But lately, I've adopted a different mindset. It's an idea of, "What if I were immortal?" I know, it sounds like I'm working on a hyperbolic chamber that promises eternal life. But trust me, I'm not that delusional.

I'm talking figuratively. The first time I got this idea was when I read one of Marcus Aurelius' Meditations:

"Think of yourself as dead. You have lived your life. Now take what's left and live properly."

I'm particularly referring to the last part: Living properly. What does that mean? I think everyone has a different perspective. To me, living properly means that I'm satisfied with my life. That I can look myself in the mirror, and genuinely say, "I like my life."

Was I truly satisfied when I lived my life in the now? No, not really. I didn't have a real career, or a house, or anything that I was proud of. And why was that? I was too focused on the now. I wanted things to happen fast.

"Before you know it, you'll be dead!" Now, that mindset is fine to get started. Nothing works better than kicking someone in the butt by telling them they're going to die.

But once you're working on building a LIFE, it's not helpful to think like that. Being present is a great thing, but like many things in life, don't overdo it.

That's why I like to live like I'm immortal. Because when you live forever…

- You have all the time in the world to build something.

- You can make mistakes and learn from them.

- There's no pressure to make things happen fast.

- You treat people with respect because other people will also be around forever.

This small tweak in my mindset has helped me to take a different view on life. I'm not afraid to look 10 or 20 years ahead. That helps me to make better decisions TODAY.

For example, I'd rather save my money or invest it instead of spending it because I know that "future Darius" will benefit from that.

"But how about the present, Darius?"

Well, I talked about being satisfied, right? Odd enough, I'm more satisfied when I SAVE my money. Or when I eat healthy food or work out every day. When I think about this idea, I find it fascinating how well it works.

We all know we're going to die (I recently even wrote an article about it). That's a good and bad thing.

- Good because it gives us urgency.
- Bad because we lose sight of the big picture.

How do you live? Like a mortal or immortal person?

Whatever it is, I hope you're *satisfied* with your life. Because at the end of the day, that's what matters most.

The Power Of Compounding: You Can Achieve Anything, If You Stop Trying To Do Everything

Do you have a long list of goals, desires, and wants for your life? Do you want to learn more? Earn more? Improve your skills? Get the most out of your relationships? Live better?

All those things are good. Life is about moving forward and making consistent progress. However, there's one important thing about all this working, hustling, striving, and achieving more: You can't do everything at the same time.

That's common sense, right? You only have so much time and energy. So if you take on too many things, you end up spread too thin. Instead, it's much more effective to focus your effort on one thing.

Success Adds Up

Real success happens when we focus on one thing at a time. The first time I discovered that idea was in high school. When I was preparing for my final exams, I decided to study only one subject at a time. And I only moved on to the next when I fully grasped the material.

I noticed that I could learn something way faster if I immersed myself in it for a few days. Most of my peers studied multiple subjects a day. I never like that approach because it's too scattered.

If I'm working on a project at work, I don't pick up another big project. If I'm working on a new course for my blog, I don't start writing a book at the same time. That strategy helps me to get things done quicker and better. Hence, I achieve much more when I give my attention to one thing.

Gary Keller and Jay Papasan, authors of The One Thing, which is a great book about this same concept, said it best:

"Where I'd had huge success, I had narrowed my concentration to one thing, and where my success varied, my focus had too."

Are you working on a lot of things? Is your attention not on one thing? There's a big chance that you will not achieve the best possible results. Or worse: You might fail if you try to achieve many things at the same time The reason is simple: Most of us believe that success happens all at once. Real life is different. Keller and Papasan put it well:

"Success is sequential, not simultaneous."

Things add up. You learn one skill. Then another. You finish one project. Then another. Over time, your accomplishments add up to form an impressive feat. This is especially true for money. Most people earned their money over time. Few people make a big financial splash. Forget about the Conor McGregors and Evan Spiegels of this world. These are people who hit the career jackpot.

But you don't need special talent or skills to succeed in life. If you take the long road, achieve one goal after the other, and build up your wealth step by step, you are more likely to live a good life. It's simple. And it always works. People who say it doesn't just haven't had the patience to apply it to their own life. One of my mentors owns a few dozen properties, worth millions. He acquired his wealth over time. He's in his sixties now. You see, things take time. And when you combine patience with compounding, you achieve the biggest results.

And these are not extraordinary things. I'm not promising you a gold medal at the 2020 Olympics or that you'll become the next Zuckerberg. *Everyone* can save money, improve their skills, and create wealth.

The Impact Of Long-Term Compounding

It's incredibly corny example, but take Warren Buffett. This is how he built his wealth over time.

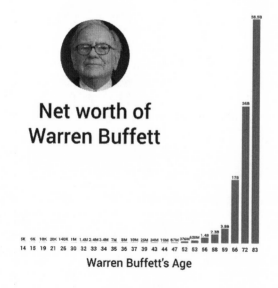

Net worth of Warren Buffett

Warren Buffett's Age

Don't look at the numbers (or random x-axis). Look at the relative growth.

Between age 32 and age 44, Buffett improved his net worth by 1257%. That's pretty exceptional growth over 12 years, right? Especially if you take into account that he lost a lot of money in his 40s. But that's not the point here.

Look at this. From age 44 to 56, Warren Buffett's wealth increased by a ridiculous 7268% over a similar time period. And of course, this is his net worth and there's always luck involved with these type of numbers. Plus, his net worth is based on stock prices — which means a big portion of it could be all gone tomorrow. But still, it's about the growth he achieved over time.

Another thing: Buffett acquired 99% of his net worth after he became 50. Think about all those spoiled idiots in their teens, twenties, and even thirties (me included), who complain about the slow progress of their career. This helps you to put things in perspective.

Anyway, there's a lot of Warren Buffett porn on the internet. And a lot of people pretend you can become rich by investing in the stock market. All you need to do is to buy their course that contains all the secrets to wealth.

Yeah right. It doesn't work that way. Personally, I hate stocks, and I think normal folks should stay away from Wall Street. I prefer real estate. However, Buffett is the perfect example of sequential success. You can achieve big things with small actions, that build up over time.

This is not only true for money. The same concept applies to skills, health, and relationships.You don't build a strong body in a day, month, or even a year. It takes years of consistent effort. Shortcuts don't exist, no matter how 'smart' you work.

For example, cyclists under the age of 28 rarely win big races like The Tour The France because it takes them years to build the strength, stamina, and mindset you need to win.

If you want to see the impact of compounding in your own life, it requires you to focus on one thing at a time (for every aspect of your life) and always look at the bigger picture.

It comes down to this: You'll get there if you put in the work. Who cares if it's tomorrow or 20 years? It *will* happen. That's all that matters.

Postscript

After spending hours of reading and editing my own articles of the past three years, I noticed that there are a lot of contradictions. I'm very pleased with that. A person who doesn't contradicts himself is an idiot.

Life is not about what you know. It's about what you don't know. And we never know enough. That's good news for the both of us. It means that until the day we die, we can keep learning.

Another thing I noticed is that I forgot about some of the things I wrote. "Did I write that?" It's not that I'm impressed by my own writing. Far from it. I'm surprised by the amount of knowledge that we forget. The good thing is that I'm aware of this human flaw. We think we know a lot because we might be well read—but in fact, we forget more than we remember.

I will keep referring back to the things I've learned, and I will never assume I've "mastered" something. Because there is always more to learn.

Thanks for reading this book.

Please let me know your thoughts. Feel free to email me on: darius@dariusforoux.com.

-Darius

Thanks For Reading

Thank you for taking the time to read this until the end. I appreciate that you decided to spend your time on this book, and not on the millions of other things that you could do. My goal with every piece of content I create is to share something I wish someone else had told me earlier.

I've committed myself to lifelong learning and I share everything on my blog and books. Without a reader, I'm not a writer. So, thank you for making me a writer.

If you want to stay in touch or write me an email, sign up to my free newsletter here: dariusforoux.com.

-Darius